Frontiers in Noninvasive Cardiac Mapping

Editors

ASHOK J. SHAH
MICHEL HAISSAGUERRE
MELEZE HOCINI

CARDIAC ELECTROPHYSIOLOGY CLINICS

www.cardiacEP.theclinics.com

Consulting Editors
RANJAN K. THAKUR
ANDREA NATALE

March 2015 • Volume 7 • Number 1

ELSEVIER

1600 John F. Kennedy Boulevard ● Suite 1800 ● Philadelphia, Pennsylvania, 19103-2899

http://www.theclinics.com

CARDIAC ELECTROPHYSIOLOGY CLINICS Volume 7, Number 1
March 2015 ISSN 1877-9182, ISBN-13: 978-0-323-35651-0

Editor: Adrianne Brigido
Developmental Editor: Barbara Cohen-Kligerman

Cardiac Electrophysiology Clinics (ISSN 1877-9182) is published quarterly by Elsevier Inc., 360 Park Avenue South, New York, NY 10010-1710. Months of issue are March, June, September, and December. Subscription prices are $200.00 per year for US individuals, $293.00 per year for US institutions, $105.00 per year for US students and residents, $225.00 per year for Canadian individuals, $331.00 per year for Canadian institutions, $285.00 per year for international individuals, $354.00 per year for international institutions and $150.00 per year for Canadian and international students/residents. To receive student/resident rate, orders must be accompanied by name of affiliated institution, date of term, and the signature of program/residency coordinator on institution letterhead. Orders will be billed at individual rate until proof of status is received. Foreign air speed delivery is included in all Clinics subscription prices. All prices are subject to change without notice. **POSTMASTER:** Send address changes to Cardiac Electrophysiology Clinics, Elsevier Health Sciences Division, Subscription Customer Service, 3251 Riverport Lane, Maryland Heights, MO 63043. **Customer Service: 1-800-654-2452 (US and Canada). From outside of the US and Canada, call 314-477-8871. Fax: 314-447-8029. E-mail:** JournalsCustomerService-usa@elsevier.com **(for print support);** JournalsOnlineSupport-usa@elsevier.com **(for online support).**

Reprints. For copies of 100 or more of articles in this publication, please contact the Commercial Reprints Department, Elsevier Inc., 360 Park Avenue South, New York, NY 10010-1710. Tel.: 212-633-3874; Fax: 212-633-3820; E-mail: reprints@elsevier.com.

Contributors

CONSULTING EDITORS

RANJAN K. THAKUR, MD, MPH, MBA, FHRS
Professor of Medicine and Director, Arrhythmia
Service, Thoracic and Cardiovascular Institute,
Sparrow Health System, Michigan State
University, Lansing, Michigan

ANDREA NATALE, MD, FACC, FHRS
Executive Medical Director, Texas Cardiac
Arrhythmia Institute, St. David's Medical
Center, Austin, Texas; Consulting Professor,
Division of Cardiology, Stanford University,
Palo Alto, California; Adjunct Professor of
Medicine, Heart and Vascular Center, Case
Western Reserve University, Cleveland, Ohio;
Director, Interventional Electrophysiology,
Scripps Clinic, San Diego, California; Senior
Clinical Director, EP Services, California
Pacific Medical Center, San Francisco,
California

EDITORS

ASHOK J. SHAH, MD
IHU LIRYC, Electrophysiology and Heart
Modeling Institute, Fondation Bordeaux
Université, Bordeaux, France

MICHEL HAISSAGUERRE, MD
IHU LIRYC, Electrophysiology and Heart
Modeling Institute, Fondation Bordeaux
Université, Bordeaux, France

MELEZE HOCINI, MD
IHU LIRYC, Electrophysiology and Heart
Modeling Institute, Fondation Bordeaux
Université, Bordeaux, France

AUTHORS

NORA ALJEFAIRI, MD
IHU LIRYC, Electrophysiology and Heart
Modeling Institute, Fondation Bordeaux
Université, Bordeaux, France

FELIPE ATIENZA, MD
Cardiology Department, Hospital General
Universitario Gregorio Marañón, Madrid,
Spain

JASON BAYER, PhD
LIRYC Electrophysiology and Heart Modelling
Institute, University of Bordeaux, Bordeaux,
France

LAURA BEAR, PhD
IHU LIRYC, Electrophysiology and
Heart Modeling Institute, Fondation
Bordeaux Université; Inserm U1045,
Cardiothoracic Research Center,
Bordeaux, France

OMER BERENFELD, PhD, FHRS
Center for Arrhythmia Research, University of
Michigan, Ann Arbor, Michigan

OLIVIER BERNUS, PhD
IHU LIRYC, Electrophysiology and Heart
Modeling Institute, Fondation Bordeaux
Université; Inserm U1045, Cardiothoracic
Research Center, Bordeaux, France

BENJAMIN BERTE, MD
IHU LIRYC, Electrophysiology and Heart
Modeling Institute, Fondation Bordeaux
Université, Bordeaux, France

PIERRE BORDACHAR, MD, PhD
CHU Bordeaux, LIRYC Institute Bordeaux,
Université de Bordeaux, France

IVAN CAKULEV, MD
Division of Cardiovascular Medicine,
Department of Medicine, Harrington Heart &
Vascular Institute, University Hospitals Case
Medical Center, Cleveland, Ohio

RICHARD H. CLAYTON, PhD
Insigneo Institute for *in-silico* Medicine,
Department of Computer Science, University
of Sheffield, Sheffield, United Kingdom

ANDREU M. CLIMENT, PhD
Cardiology Department, Hospital General
Universitario Gregorio Marañón, Madrid,
Spain

PHILLIP S. CUCULICH, MD
Cardiovascular Diseases and
Electrophysiology, Barnes-Jewish Hospital,
Washington University School of Medicine,
St Louis, Missouri

ARNAUD DENIS, MD
IHU LIRYC, Electrophysiology and Heart
Modeling Institute, Fondation Bordeaux
Université, Bordeaux, France

NICOLAS DERVAL, MD
IHU LIRYC, Electrophysiology and Heart
Modeling Institute, Fondation Bordeaux
Université, Bordeaux, France

AMIT DOSHI, MD
Cardiac Electrophysiolgist, Division of
Cardiac Electrophysiology, Mercy
Heart & Vascular Center, St Louis, St Louis,
Missouri

RÉMI DUBOIS, PhD
IHU LIRYC, Electrophysiology and Heart
Modeling Institute, Fondation Bordeaux
Université; Inserm U1045, Cardiothoracic
Research Center, Bordeaux, France

JEROME EDWARDS, BS, MBA
CardioNXT, Inc, Westminster, Colorado

IGOR EFIMOV, PhD
IHU LIRYC, Electrophysiology and Heart
Modeling Institute, Fondation Bordeaux
Université, Bordeaux, France; Professor,
Department of Biomedical Engineering,
Washington University School of Medicine,
Washington University in St Louis, St Louis,
Missouri

DAMIR ERKAPIC, MD
Consultant in Electrophysiology, Medical
Clinic I, Department of Cardiology, Justus-
Liebig University of Giessen, Giessen,
Germany

SABINE ERNST, MD, FESC
Department of Cardiology, Royal Brompton
Hospital; Consultant Cardiologist/
Electrophysiologist, Reader Cardiology,
NIHR Cardiovascular Biomedical
Research Unit, Royal Brompton and
Harefield Hospital, National Heart and
Lung Institute, Imperial College London,
London, United Kingdom

ROMAIN ESCHALIER, MD, PhD
CHU Bordeaux, LIRYC Institute Bordeaux,
Université de Bordeaux, France

FEDERICO GOMEZ, MD
Department of Cardiology, Royal Brompton
Hospital, London, United Kingdom

MARÍA S. GUILLEM, PhD
Bio-ITACA, Universitat Politècnica de València,
Valencia, Spain

MICHEL HAISSAGUERRE, MD
IHU LIRYC, Electrophysiology and Heart
Modeling Institute, Fondation Bordeaux
Université, Bordeaux, France

MELEZE HOCINI, MD
IHU LIRYC, Electrophysiology and Heart
Modeling Institute, Fondation Bordeaux
Université, Bordeaux, France

DARREN HOOKS, MBChB
IHU LIRYC, Electrophysiology and Heart
Modeling Institute, Fondation Bordeaux
Université, Bordeaux, France

PIERRE JAIS, MD
Clinical Professor, Department of Cardiology, Division of Rhythmology and Cardiac Stimulation, Hôpital Cardiologique du Haut-Lévêque and Université de Bordeaux, Institut LIRYC, Bordeaux, France

AJIT H. JANARDHAN, MD, PhD
CardioNXT, Inc, Westminster, Colorado

PRAPA KANAGARATNAM, MA, MBBChir, MRCP, PhD
Consultant in Cardiology and Electrophysiology, Department of Cardiac Electrophysiology, Hammersmith & St Mary's Hospitals, Imperial College Healthcare NHS Trust, London, United Kingdom

PAUL KESSMAN, BS
CardioNXT, Inc, Westminster, Colorado

THOMAS KURIAN, MD
Cardiac Electrophysiolgist, Division of Cardiac Electrophysiology, Mercy Heart & Vascular Center, St Louis, St Louis, Missouri

KEVIN MING WEI LEONG, MBBS, MRCP
Clinical Electrophysiology Research Fellow, Faculty of Medicine, National Heart & Lung Institute, Imperial College London, United Kingdom

HAN S. LIM, MBBS, PhD
IHU LIRYC, Electrophysiology and Heart Modeling Institute, Fondation Bordeaux Université, Bordeaux, France

PHANG BOON LIM, MA, MBBChir, MRCP, PhD
Consultant in Cardiology and Electrophysiology, Department of Cardiac Electrophysiology, Hammersmith and St Mary's Hospitals, Imperial College Healthcare NHS Trust, London, United Kingdom

BRUCE D. LINDSAY, MD
Section Head, Clinical Cardiac Electrophysiology, Cardiovascular Medicine, Cleveland Clinic Foundation, Cleveland, Ohio

SAAGAR MAHIDA, MBChB
IHU LIRYC, Electrophysiology and Heart Modeling Institute, Fondation Bordeaux Université, Bordeaux, France

LILIAN MANTZIARI, MD
Department of Cardiology, Royal Brompton Hospital, London, United Kingdom

VALENTIN MEILLET, MSc
LIRYC Electrophysiology and Heart Modelling Institute, University of Bordeaux; INSERM U1045, Cardiothoracic Research Center, Bordeaux, France

MARTYN P. NASH, PhD
Auckland Bioengineering Institute and Engineering Science, University of Auckland, Auckland, New Zealand

THOMAS NEUMANN, MD
Professor, Department of Cardiology, Kerckhoff Heart and Thorax Center, Bad Nauheim, Germany

BAO NGUYEN, BS
CardioNXT, Inc, Westminster, Colorado

ALI PASHAEI, PhD
LIRYC Electrophysiology and Heart Modelling Institute, University of Bordeaux; INSERM U1045, Cardiothoracic Research Center, Bordeaux, France

STEPHEN PIEPER, MD
Cardiac Electrophysiolgist, Division of Cardiac Electrophysiology, Mercy Heart & Vascular Center, St Louis, St Louis, Missouri

SYLVAIN PLOUX, MD, PhD
CHU Bordeaux, LIRYC Institute Bordeaux, Université de Bordeaux, France

PHILIPPE RITTER, MD
CHU Bordeaux, LIRYC Institute Bordeaux, Université de Bordeaux, France

KARINE ROY, MD
Department of Cardiology, Royal Brompton Hospital, London, United Kingdom

YORAM RUDY, PhD
Director of the Cardiac Bioelectricity and Arrhythmia Center (CBAC); The Fred Saigh Distinguished Professor, Washington University, St Louis, Missouri

RIIKKA RYDMAN, MD
Department of Cardiology, Royal Brompton Hospital, London, United Kingdom

FRÉDÉRIC SACHER, MD
IHU LIRYC, Electrophysiology and Heart
Modeling Institute, Fondation Bordeaux
Université, Bordeaux, France

JOHAN SAENEN, MD
Department of Cardiology, Royal Brompton
Hospital, London, United Kingdom

JAYAKUMAR SAHADEVAN, MD
Department of Cardiology, Louis Stokes
Cleveland Veterans Affairs Medical Center,
Cleveland, Ohio

MAURICIO SANCHEZ, MD
Cardiac Electrophysiolgist, Division of
Cardiac Electrophysiology, Mercy Heart &
Vascular Center, St Louis, St Louis, Missouri

ASHOK J. SHAH, MD
IHU LIRYC, Electrophysiology and Heart
Modeling Institute, Fondation Bordeaux
Université, Bordeaux, France

JENNIFER N.A. SILVA, MD
Director, Pediatric Electrophsyiology; Assistant
Professor, Pediatrics, Division of Pediatric
Cardiology, Saint Louis Children's Hospital,
Washington University School of Medicine,
St Louis, Missouri

IRINA SUMAN-HORDUNA, MD
Department of Cardiology, Royal Brompton
Hospital, London, United Kingdom

NIRAJ VARMA, MD, PhD, FRCP
Cleveland Clinic, Cleveland, Ohio

EDWARD VIGMOND, PhD
LIRYC Electrophysiology and Heart Modelling
Institute, University of Bordeaux, Bordeaux,
France; Bordeaux Institute of Mathematics,
University of Bordeaux, Talence, France

ALBERT L. WALDO, MD, PhD (Hon)
Division of Cardiovascular Medicine,
Department of Medicine, Harrington Heart &
Vascular Institute, University Hospitals Case
Medical Center, Cleveland, Ohio

BRUCE WILKOFF, MD
Cleveland Clinic, Cleveland, Ohio

SEIGO YAMASHITA, MD
IHU LIRYC, Electrophysiology and Heart
Modeling Institute, Fondation Bordeaux
Université, Bordeaux, France

STEPHAN ZELLERHOFF, MD
IHU LIRYC, Electrophysiology and Heart
Modeling Institute, Fondation Bordeaux
Université, Bordeaux, France

Contents

understanding of the underlying pathophysiologic processes of this common heart rhythm disorder.

detailed characterization of electrical substrate and its interaction with pacing. Electrocardiogram (ECG) features affect CRT outcomes. However, the surface ECG reports rudimentary electrical data. In contrast, noninvasive electrocardiographic imaging provides high-resolution single-beat ventricular mapping. Several complex characteristics of electrical substrate, not decipherable from the 12-lead ECG, are linked to CRT effect. CRT response may be improved by candidate selection and left ventricular lead placement directed by more precise electrical evaluation, on an individual patient basis.

Noninvasive electrocardiographic imaging (ECGI) has been used in pediatric and congenital heart patients to better understand their electrophysiologic substrates. In this article we focus on the 4 subjects related to pediatric ECGI: (1) ECGI in patients with congenital heart disease and Wolff–Parkinson–White syndrome, (2) ECGI in patients with hypertrophic cardiomyopathy and preexcitation, (3) ECGI in pediatric patients with Wolff–Parkinson–White syndrome, and (4) ECGI for pediatric cardiac resynchronization therapy.

Noninvasive mapping overcomes previous barriers to provide panoramic beat-to-beat mapping during atrial fibrillation (AF). This article demonstrates the utility of noninvasive mapping in identifying localized driving sources in persistent AF. Reentrant driver activity detected by noninvasive mapping from specific regions correlated with distinct f-wave morphologies. Ablation targeting these drivers resulted in progressive AF cycle length prolongation and termination of the arrhythmia.

Recent clinical trials using panoramic mapping techniques have shown success in targeting rotors and focal impulses in atrial fibrillation (AF). Ablations directed toward these organized sources improve outcomes in AF. The left atrial appendage (LAA) has been suspected as a possible extrapulmonary source of AF, and ablation within the LAA or electrical isolation of the LAA improves outcomes in certain cases. This case highlights a unique example of panoramic imaging created with a computational mapping algorithm integrated in 3-dimensional mapping, which identified rotors within the LAA. Furthermore, ablations performed near an identified rotor core within the LAA terminated AF.

CARDIAC ELECTROPHYSIOLOGY CLINICS

Foreword

Noninvasive Cardiac Mapping: A New Era in Electrophysiology

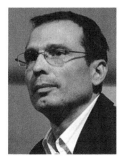

Pierre Jais, MD

Medical doctors have long dreamed of directly seeing the inside of the human body to diagnose a patient's clinical problem and visualize the underlying pathologic abnormality. While imaging partly realized the "en direct" visualization goal in several fields of medicine, in electrophysiology (EP), the information continued to be available indirectly through cardiac signatures inscribed on 12-lead electrocardiogram (ECG) paper. Electrocardiographic technique did not evolve much for a century since the time that Waller and Einthoven pioneered it. Interestingly, the noninvasive mapping technique developed by the team of Yoram Rudy inverts body surface electrocardiographic information gathered from 250 chest electrodes, and, in combination with the imaging data, provides detailed and spatially resolved electrical 3D mapping of the heart. Rudy's team researched complex mathematics to solve the arduous inverse problem (getting from the surface of the chest back to the heart). While many necessary improvements will, no doubt, happen in the future, this pioneering effort has paved the way for a new era in cardiac EP.

The current applications of this technique covered in this issue of *Cardiac Electrophysiology Clinics* nicely illustrate how wide the field is, and give a flavor of how much it can grow. The initial application to localize focal ventricular arrhythmias such as ventricular premature beats was probably the easiest to challenge and validates the concept. An encouraging spatial resolution of 6 mm was demonstrated, and challenging locations at right and left ventricular outflow tracts were successfully identified. This information complemented the conventional 12-lead ECG and allowed for easier and faster ablation procedures. The same applied for difficult accessory pathways. But the real challenge for this technology was fibrillating rhythms, particularly from the atria, where the signal at the level of torso is weak compared with that from the ventricles. Looking at the noninvasive activation maps recorded in atrial fibrillation (AF) was initially disappointing if not discouraging. But with this kind of tool that provides a panoramic (of all heart chambers) electromap of fibrillating atria, it was possible to phase analyze the electrical signals as do basic EP scientists who have been experimenting for decades with optical signals acquired using voltage-sensitive contrast agents (optical mapping) during in vitro atrial/ventricular fibrillation. Despite significant challenges and reasons for failure, it did work, and the recently demonstrated impact on AF ablation is both a proof of concept

Card Electrophysiol Clin 7 (2015) xiii–xiv
http://dx.doi.org/10.1016/j.ccep.2014.12.001

cardiacEP.theclinics.com

and a major procedural improvement for patients. In heart failure due to electrical conduction disorders and resynchronization therapy, investigators have shown encouraging clinical observations that need randomized studies to establish this mapping strategy as a key player. Initial work on ventricular fibrillation and repolarization mapping reveals fascinating characteristics unseen before. Thus, finally, the management of 3 major epidemics—AF, heart failure, and sudden cardiac death—will continue to benefit from this mapping technology, which promises to open a new era in our field.

Pierre Jais, MD
Department of Cardiology
Division of Rhythmology and Cardiac Stimulation
Hôpital Cardiologique du Haut-Lévêque
Avenue de Magellan
33604 Bordeaux-Pessac, France

E-mail address:
pierre.jais@chu-bordeaux.fr

Introduction to Noninvasive Cardiac Mapping

Laura Bear, PhD[a,b], Phillip S. Cuculich, MD[c,*,1],
Olivier Bernus, PhD[a,b], Igor Efimov, PhD[a,d],
Rémi Dubois, PhD[a,b,1]

KEYWORDS

● Electrocardiogram ● Inverse solution ● Forward problem ● Mapping

KEY POINTS

- The need for more precise, noninvasive evaluation of cardiac electrophysiology has driven the development of inverse-solution-based methods.
- The ultimate goal is to accurately calculate potentials on the surface of the heart using measured potentials from the body surface. This requires 2 steps: (1) the forward solution—development of a mathematical construct describing the potential field throughout the torso and on the body surface as a function of the epicardial potentials and (2) the inverse solution—inversion of this formulation to calculate potentials on the epicardial surface as measured from the body surface.
- The forward solution makes use of numerical methods, such as boundary element method or method of fundamental solutions.
- The inverse solution is subject to large noise-related errors (the problem is ill posed); to address these noise-related errors, regularization methods have been developed and validated, including the Tikhonov and generalized minimal residual (GMRes) methods.
- Extensive testing and validation of the mathematic methods has occurred in several highly controlled experiments, including torso tank models and human intraoperative mapping.

INTRODUCTION

A 55-year-old man develops crushing chest pain and presents to an emergency room for evaluation. In the first few minutes, a single test is performed that accurately diagnoses the problem and the man urgently undergoes a life-saving procedure...

A 20-year-old young woman complains of sustained palpitations and near syncope. In the clinic, she undergoes a single test that accurately diagnoses the problem and the woman undergoes a procedure that cures her palpitations...

An 80-year-old woman is admitted to the hospital with a history of recurrent unexplained embolic

Disclosure: This work was supported through the Investment of the Future grant, ANR-10-IAHU-04, from the government of France through the Agence National de la Recherche. Rémi Dubois, PhD is paid consultant and is stockowners in CardioInsight Inc.

a IHU LIRYC, Electrophysiology and Heart Modeling Institute, Fondation Bordeaux Université, Bordeaux, France; b Inserm U1045, Cardiothoracic Research Center, 146 rue Léo-Saignat, Bordeaux Cedex 33076, France; c Cardiovascular Diseases and Electrophysiology, Barnes-Jewish Hospital, Washington University School of Medicine, 660 South Euclid Avenue, Campus Box 8086, St Louis, MO 63110, USA; d Department of Biomedical Engineering, Washington University School of Medicine, 390E Whitaker Hall, One Brookings Drive, St. Louis, MO 63130, USA

1 Shared senior authors.
* Corresponding author.
E-mail address: pcuculic@wustl.edu

strokes. She undergoes a single test that identifies a potential source for the embolic strokes, and blood thinner treatment is initiated to dramatically reduce her risk of future events…

In each of these cases, and in millions more like these worldwide each year, the electrocardiogram (ECG) helps physicians rapidly come to cardiac diagnoses and confidently initiate treatment plans. As such, the ECG has become ubiquitous in clinical medicine and is a cornerstone in nearly all studies of cardiovascular diseases.

The original 3-lead ECG was developed more than 100 years ago. Nevertheless, ECG remains relevant today because of its gradual evolution to higher resolution ECG culminating into a truly transformative development of ECG Imaging. Very few useful technologies, especially in health care, survive for so long.[1] The durable technologies that advance seem to blend the initial physiologic principles with computerized modernization. For example, in the late nineteenth century, around the time of the early development of the ECG, Wilhelm Röentgen discovered the X-ray. Over the course of the next century, noninvasive imaging of the heart's structure rapidly moved from Röentgen's 2-dimensional imaging of a stationary cardiac silhouette to the millimeter precision of advanced three-dimensional (3D) and 4-dimensional imaging modalities such as echocardiography, computed tomography (CT), and magnetic resonance (MR) imaging.

Compared with structural imaging, advances in noninvasive imaging of cardiac electrophysiology have largely lagged. However, in the past several decades, there has been tremendous growth in clinical cardiac electrophysiology, especially driven by invasive catheter mapping and therapies. This growth has fueled both the clinical and research needs for more precise understanding of cardiac electrophysiology that extends beyond the traditional ECG. This article outlines the important progress from ECG development, through more extensive measurement of body surface potentials, and the fundamental leap to solving the inverse problem of electrocardiography, with a focus on mathematical methods and experimental validation.

DEVELOPMENT OF THE ELECTROCARDIOGRAM

Cardiac electrical activity produces currents that propagate through the torso and onto the skin surface, where they can be recorded as an ECG. One of the first reported recordings of an ECG was made by British physiologist, Augustus D. Waller, using a Lippmann capillary electrometer.[2,3] Willem Einthoven further developed the ECG using a string galvanometer,[4] producing high-quality waveforms comparable to those used today. As this invention was before the development of self-adhesive electrodes, ECGs were recorded by submersing the hands and feet of a subject in saline-filled buckets, allowing a large contact area with the skin (**Fig. 1**). Hence, the standard limb lead system was developed, defined as the voltage difference between the recordings on each arm and the left leg.

The ECG was further extended with the development of the precordial unipolar lead system,[5] allowing the electrical activity of the heart to be viewed in the horizontal plane. Six electrodes (V_1 through V_6) are placed on the chest, directly over the heart (**Fig. 2**). Rather than taking the difference between 2 chest electrodes like the standard bipolar limb leads, potentials are referenced to the Wilson's central terminal (WCT), approximating a zero reference potential.[6] The WCT led to the development of the augmented limb leads, aVR, aVL, and aVF.[7] These leads modify the standard limb leads by referencing to the WCT. The precordial, augmented, and standard limb lead systems combine to form the standard 12-lead ECG used today (**Fig. 3**).

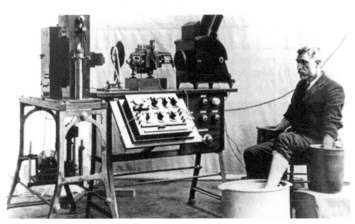

Fig. 1. The first practical electrocardiogram using a string galvanometer recorded from the subject's limbs immersed in containers of saline solution. (*From* Barron SL. The development of the electrocardiograph in Great Britain. Br Med J 1950;1(4655):720–5.)

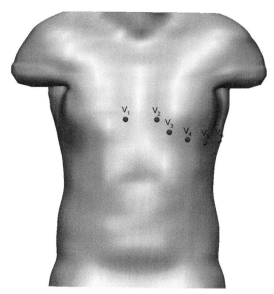

Fig. 2. Electrode placement for the precordial lead system (numbered V_1 through V_6 from left to right), concentrated over the heart. Additional electrodes are also placed on the left and right arms and the left leg for the standard 12-lead ECG. (Model *courtesy of* The Auckland Bioengineering Institute, Auckland, New Zealand; with permission.)

ADDRESSING LIMITATIONS OF THE ELECTROCARDIOGRAM: BODY SURFACE POTENTIAL MAPPING

The standard 12-lead ECG is limited by the scarcity of spatial information, preventing the precise localization of abnormal electrical events.[8,9] Body surface potential mapping (BSPM) uses additional leads to record potentials from broad areas of the torso (between 32 and 256), which can be visualized temporally as 3D maps (**Fig. 4**). The additional recording sites can capture information missed by the standard 12-lead ECG, producing a more complete picture of the underlying cardiac electrical activity.

BSPM has been used in both experimental and clinical setting for the detection and diagnosis of various pathologic conditions. Previous studies have demonstrated its utility in identifying patients at risk of recurrent sustained ventricular arrhythmias,[10,11] improving the detection of acute and chronic myocardial infarction,[12,13] noninvasively characterizing reentrant ventricular tachycardia (VT),[14,15] and, more recently, localizing maximal frequency sites in atrial fibrillation.[16]

The ability to determine precise details of cardiac electrical activity from BSPM is limited by the filtering effects of the torso cavity, that is, body surface potentials are a smoothed representation of the underlying global cardiac electrical activity. Over time, the incremental advances of BSPM over traditional 12-lead ECG have not justified the additional procedural complexity, inconsistent interpretations, or increased expense that accompanies these methods.

Direct mapping of cardiac potentials provides signals that have not been modified or smoothed by passing through the torso volume. This mapping is typically achieved percutaneously using a

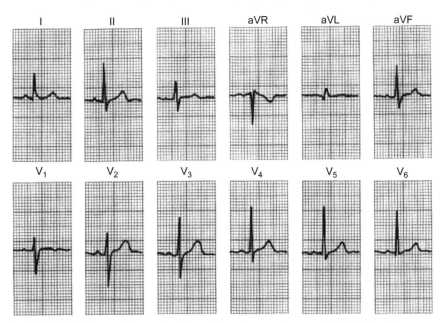

Fig. 3. Standard 12-lead ECG traces from a healthy subject (I, II, and III, standard limb leads; aVR, aVL, and aVF, augmented limb leads; and V_1 through V_6, precordial leads).

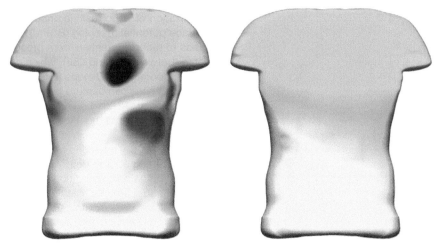

Fig. 4. Body surface potential distribution at the peak of the R-wave during sinus rhythm. Potentials are displayed on a realistic human torso model with anterior (*left*) and posterior (*right*) views. Positive potentials are represented in red and negative in blue. (Model *courtesy of* The Auckland Bioengineering Institute, Auckland, New Zealand; with permission.)

roving catheter[17,18] or a multielectrode noncontact catheter.[19–21] However, these techniques are invasive and cannot be used for long-term monitoring. Furthermore, catheter-based mapping tools are generally limited to characterizing endocardial activity, potentially missing information about intramural activation pathways in reentrant circuits. Accurate mapping also requires consistent and reproducible catheter contact, which can be time consuming. A different approach to understanding cardiac electrophysiology is to transform body surface potentials mathematically, removing the smoothing effect of the torso volume and reconstructing the cardiac source directly. These global maps of cardiac electrophysiology may provide further information about intramural breakthrough and epicardial exit sites. This information would allow better understanding of the critical elements necessary to initiate and maintain tachycardia and could also be used to aid in interventional clinical cardiac electrophysiology by addressing some of the shortcomings of catheter mapping.

MOVING INWARD: INVERSE SOLUTION ELECTROCARDIOGRAPHY

A more useful imaging modality would provide accurate information about local myocardial potential distribution on the heart using information obtained from BSPM. The inverse problem of electrocardiography seeks to noninvasively reconstruct cardiac electrical activity from remote body surface measurements. However, mathematically and technically, this can be challenging. The numerical solution for the inverse computation requires 2 steps: (1) the forward problem—a

mathematical construct that expresses the potential distribution across the body surface and throughout the torso volume conductor, as a function of the cardiac source, and (2) the inverse problem—transposition of the forward problem to compute the cardiac source from the measured torso potential data. Despite the conceptual simplicity of the forward problem, the inversion of this relationship to solve the inverse problem is far from trivial. Even when a unique solution exists, the inverse problem is often ill posed, meaning that small levels of noise become exponentially amplified. To overcome this, regularized solutions to the inverse problem have been developed.

Cardiac Source Model

The formulation of the forward model begins with the cardiac source description. Initial investigations often approximated the cardiac source as either single or multiple equivalent dipoles.[22,23] However, these models are limited by being equivalent entities. That is, there are no obvious physical or physiologic links between these models and the true sources they represent, or any directly measurable quantities. Cardiac potential and myocardial activation sequences are currently the most common source models used in forward and inverse studies.[24–27] Potential-based models represent the cardiac source using extracellular potentials on the heart surface, whereas myocardial activation time models use the time of activation. Activation times are described as the time of arrival of the depolarization phase of an action potential and can be defined either through the 3D myocardial wall or on the heart surface including both the epicardium and endocardium.

One benefit of potential-based models is that extracellular potentials are measurable quantities. Activation times must be derived from recorded electrograms or optical signals. Moreover, although activation times can be derived from extracellular potentials, the reverse is not true. That is, the additional information contained within a potential distribution, such as repolarization and recovery processes, are not available with activation times. On the other hand, whereas potential-based models can provide information on both epicardial and endocardial surfaces,[28] activation-based models theoretically can provide direct information about transmural propagation.

Forward Problem Formulation

Once the cardiac source is defined, the governing equations defining the potential distribution within the torso can be derived. These equations are numerically solved over the volume conductor within which the source is located. Although the mathematical formulation of the relationship between the heart and body surface potentials is different, the final system of equations is the same regardless of the cardiac source model used. This system is a standard linear system:

$$\phi_T = A\phi_H \tag{1}$$

where A is the transfer matrix, φ_H is the vector describing the cardiac source (ie, the cardiac potential field on the heat surface), and φ_T is the vector of body surface potentials (cardiac potential field on the torso).

Governing equations

The potential distribution within the torso volume conductor (**Fig. 5**) can be described by Maxwell equations. These equations relate electric and magnetic fields to their sources, charge density,

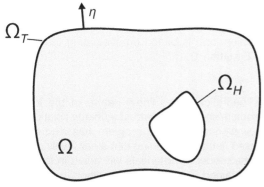

Fig. 5. A transverse slice through the torso. Shown from the center are the epicardial surface, Ω_H; the torso volume, Ω; and the skin surface, Ω_T, where η is the outward normal direction.

and current density. Cardiac electrical activity is the predominant source defining body surface potentials. Extensive testing has demonstrated that the torso volume conductor has negligible capacitive and inductive effects. The torso is essentially resistive in nature.[29–31] Furthermore, it is assumed that the electric events can be described independent of time. That is, they are static: charges are fixed or move in a steady flow. Therefore, a quasi-static assumption is used[32] allowing the torso to be approximated as a passive volume conductor. Under these conditions, the electric field density within the torso, E, is defined as:

$$E = -\nabla\varphi \tag{2}$$

where φ is the electrical potential field. In any region of the torso volume, the total electric current density, J, is described as the sum of any current source, J_s, and the conduction current, σE, where σ is the conductivity of the tissue. Owing to the conservation of current within the torso volume, the divergence of J is equal to 0. Therefore:

$$\nabla \cdot J = \nabla \cdot (J_s + \sigma E) = 0 \Rightarrow -\nabla \cdot J_s = \nabla \cdot \sigma E \tag{3}$$

Substituting Equation 3 into 2 results in the Poisson equation:

$$\nabla \cdot (\sigma \nabla \varphi) = -\nabla \cdot J_s = I_v \tag{4}$$

where I_v is the current per unit volume in the bounded volume domain Ω.

Epicardial potential model

For an epicardial potential cardiac source, the epicardium is defined as an external boundary of the heart. Under the assumption of a source-free torso (ie, $J_s = 0$) Equation 4 becomes:

$$\nabla \cdot (\sigma \nabla \varphi) = 0 \ in \ \Omega \tag{5}$$

where Ω is the volume between the epicardial and torso surfaces (see **Fig. 5**). Therefore, the governing equation for the epicardial-potential-based forward problem is a generalized Laplace equation.

Activation-time-based model

In order to derive the governing equation for the activation-based forward problem, a standard approach is to model the electrical activity within the myocardium from which the activation times are derived. The basis of this formulation is a mathematical model of the electrical properties of cardiac muscle known as the bidomain source model,[33] which is a continuum model, representing groups of cells as discrete points with distinct intracellular and extracellular spaces. Previous models have included heart surface transmembrane potentials[34] or the spatial distribution of current dipoles.[35,36] These models can be derived from the activation patterns of the heart, which are then linearly related to the body surface potentials. The model parameters can then be iteratively adjusted in an attempt to minimize the dissimilarity between measured and heart-model-generated body surface potentials.

Boundary conditions

In addition to the propagation equations, the potential distribution must meet additional restraints. For example, at any boundary within the torso (eg, between the fat and muscle layers), interface conditions are applied ensuring that the continuity of potentials and normal current flow is maintained across the shared boundary. That is, for volumes A and B, the boundary conditions are:

$$\phi_A = \phi_B$$
$$(\sigma_A \nabla \phi_A) \cdot \eta_A = (\sigma_B \nabla \phi_B) \cdot \eta_B \qquad [6]$$

In the case of homogenous propagation, only the boundary between the heart surface and torso volume, and between the torso volume and body surface, are taken into account. As air usually surrounds the body surface, applying Equation 6 to the torso surface leads to the so-called zero flux boundary condition normal to the body surface:

$$\sigma \nabla \varphi \cdot \eta = 0 \text{ on } \Omega_T \qquad [7]$$

where η is the outward normal direction and Ω_T is the torso surface. On the heart surface Ω_H, the continuity of the potentials gives:

$$\varphi = \varphi_H (x) \text{ on } x \in \Omega_H \qquad [8]$$

where x are points located on the heart surface and φ_H are the potentials on the heart surface. In addition, a reference point y_r on the torso is usually chosen to set the potentials:

$$\varphi (y_r) = \varphi_T (y_r) = 0 \text{ on } y_r \in \Omega_T \qquad [9]$$

In conclusion, the following system of equations leads to the forward problem for a homogenous torso:

$$\nabla \cdot (\sigma \nabla \phi) = 0 \text{ in } \Omega$$
$$\sigma \nabla \phi \cdot \eta = 0 \text{ on } \Omega_T$$
$$\phi(x) = \phi_H \text{ for all } x \in \Omega_H \qquad [10]$$
$$\phi(y_r) = \phi_T(y_r) = 0 \text{ on } y_r \in \Omega_T$$

When a bidomain source model is used for the activation-based forward problem, additional equations are required to expand the previous system.

Numerical solution methods

The finite element and boundary element methods are the main methods used for numerically solving the governing equations of the forward problem over the irregular geometry of a heart-torso volume conductor. These methods simplify complex continuous problems by breaking down the larger solution domain into smaller discrete components or elements. The solution can then be found for all points within the solution domain by interpolating over the discretized subdomains through the use of basis functions.

Both the finite element and boundary element methods have their advantages and limitations. Whereas the finite element method can easily model anisotropic, inhomogeneous regions, the conductivity within a boundary element torso model is limited to being either fully isotropic or piecewise constant. However, a finite element volume conductor is discretized using volumetric meshes,[37] whereas the boundary element method uses only surface descriptions, which means that significantly fewer nodes are used and the problem can be solved with greater computational efficiency.[38] An alternative coupled approach uses the most advantageous method for each region of the torso.[39,40] This use can reduce the overall size of the problem while allowing anisotropic electrical properties to be modeled. Detailed explanations on each of these methods can be found in the literature.[37–41] Because of the simplicity of only requiring discretization of the heart and torso surfaces in the boundary element model, it is the method of choice for most cardiac applications. A recently developed meshless method of fundamental solutions has also been implemented and tested.[42] The main advantages of this approach include elimination of the meshing and mesh optimization process, elimination of mesh-induced artifact, and elimination of complex singular integrals that must be carefully handled in boundary element models.

Inverse Problem Formulation

The inverse problem, the reconstruction of cardiac electrical activity from body surface potentials, is exactly the opposite of the forward problem and is based on evaluating the inverse of Equation 1:

$$\varphi_H = A^{-1} \varphi_T \qquad [11]$$

Theoretically, the linear nature of the forward problem should reconstruct a unique solution.[43,44] However, the inverse problem has a strong ill-posed nature,[45] meaning that small levels of noise in the model or potentials will result in large, unconstrained errors in the solution, which may bear little resemblance to the true cardiac source. As noise is always present in real-world measurements, the common solution is to regularize the problem. That is, constraints are imposed on the solution spatially and/or temporally in order to obtain a realistic outcome.

The transfer matrix defined in Equation 1 is typically defined independent of time, meaning each time instant of a temporally varying potential distribution can be solved for separately, giving:

$$\phi_H = A^{\dagger}_{\lambda_t} \phi_T \qquad [12]$$

where $A^{\dagger}_{\lambda_t}$ is the regularized inverse matrix at time t. Although the transfer matrix is typically time invariant, the regularized inverse need not be. The challenge then lies in determining the type and amount of regularization to apply. Although the most commonly used method of regularization for ill-posed problems is the Tikhonov regularization (described in the following section), a large number of alternative methods are in existence today such as the GMRes method.

Tikhonov regularization

Tikhonov regularization obtains a solution to the inverse problem by minimizing the following objective function F in a least squares sense[46]:

$$F = \|A\phi_H - \phi_T\|^2_2 + \lambda^2_t \|R\phi_H\|^2_2 \qquad [13]$$

The first term is the least squares solution to Equation 1, and the second term defines a spatial constraint on the solution depending on the choice of the regularization operator, R. The choice of R determines the order of the system: zero order where R is the identity matrix (R = I) constraining the amplitude of the solution, first order where R is the surface gradient (R = G) constraining the potential gradient, and second order where R is the surface Laplacian (R = L) constraining the surface curvature in the spatial domain. The constant weighing term, λ_t, at time t controls the level of regularization, and this leads to the following regularized inverse matrix:

$$A^{\dagger}_{\lambda_t} = \left(A^T A + \lambda^2_t R^T R\right)^{-1} A^T \qquad [14]$$

This matrix can be substituted into Equation 12 to solve for epicardial potentials.

Using an analytical eccentric sphere model, Rudy and Messinger-Rapport[23] have shown that the zero-order Tikhonov regularization method performs as well as higher-order schemes. Using the zero-order Tikhonov method, Equation 12 can be written as:

$$\phi_H = \left(A^T A + \lambda^2_t I\right)^{-1} A^T \phi_T \qquad [15]$$

Regularization parameter estimation

It has been shown that the degree of regularization (ie, the value of λ_t) is critical to the accuracy of an inverse solution.[47] When regularization is too high, overdamped solutions are produced, whereas insufficient regularization results in overly noisy solutions. The most commonly accepted methods for determining the regularization parameter test several values and pick one based on some criterion.[48-51]

One of the most common approaches is the L-curve method,[26,52,53] developed by Hansen and O'Leary.[50] With this method, a log-log scale plot is created of the regularization objective function ($R\varphi_H$) against the corresponding residual objective function ($A\varphi_H - \varphi_T$) for all valid regularization parameters (λ_t).

When uncorrelated Gaussian noise in the body surface potentials dominates correlated geometric noise, the plot takes on a characteristic L-shape, as illustrated in **Fig. 6**. The optimal value for λ_t is then defined as the corner of this L-curve, or the point of maximum curvature. This point provides a balance between the residual norm and the level of regularization. However, the introduction of high-quality recording systems has led to body surface potentials with low levels of Gaussian noise, resulting in flatter curves often with no definitive point of highest curvature.

The composite residual and smoothing operator (CRESO) criterion, proposed by Colli-Franzone and colleagues[48] does not have this limitation. This method finds the regularization parameter that maximizes the difference between the derivative of the smoothing term and the derivative of the

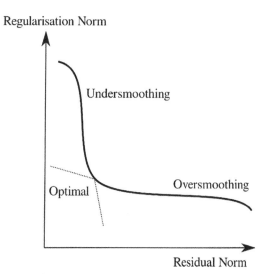

Fig. 6. The L-curve is a log-log plot of the residual norm, log $\|A\phi_H - \phi_T\|^2_2$, against the regularization norm, log $\|R\phi_H\|^2_2$. The corner of the "L" strikes a balance between the residual of the solution and the regularization norm.

residual term, that is, the smallest value of λ_t that produces the relative maximum of:

$$C(\lambda_t) = \|\phi_H\|_2^2 + 2\lambda_t^2 \frac{d}{d\lambda_t}\|\phi_H\|_2^2 \qquad [16]$$

where the function $C(\lambda_t)$ is the derivative of the function:

$$B(\lambda_t) = \lambda_t^2\|\phi_H\|_2^2 - \|A\phi_H - \phi_T\|_2^2 \qquad [17]$$

This method has shown improvements over the L-curve method in the presence of both geometric and measurement noise[51] and is commonly used in the literature.[27,42,54]

GMRes method

It is known that Tikhonov regularization can sometimes reduce spatial resolution by oversmoothing the solution. The accuracy of this regularization also depends on a priori knowledge of solution characteristics and the determination of an optimal regularization parameter. Methods to determine the regularization parameter, such as the CRESO and the L-curve method described above, may not perform consistently. To address these shortcomings, the GMRes method has been developed, which does not apply such constraints.[55–57] When compared, the accuracy of GMRes solutions was similar to that of Tikhonov regularization.[56] However, in certain cases, GMRes recovered localized potential features, which were lost with the Tikhonov solution, such as multiple potential minima.

VALIDATION STUDIES

Although forward and inverse problems are based on mathematically sound formulations, it is necessary to validate these techniques before noninvasive electrical imaging can be used routinely in a clinical setting. Numerous studies have been conducted to assess the accuracy and sensitivity of both forward and inverse solutions, and most of these have been based on computational simulations. Eccentric sphere models[22,29,30] and anatomically realistic models[58,59] have provided a framework for initial validation of different numerical methods and inverse algorithms, and this has further led to the development of several fundamental hypotheses about the effect of torso geometry and conductivity[60–62] as well as other data uncertainties on solution accuracy.[52] However, the capacity of computational methods to replicate in vivo conditions is limited.

Physical analogues have helped investigators to better understand the relationship between the cardiac source and resulting potentials and currents within the torso volume conductor.[63,64] A torso tank model with isolated heart preparation originally devised by Nagata[64] provided an experimental in vitro platform (**Fig. 7**). In these experiments, a model of a torso was filled with electrolytic solution and a perfused beating canine heart was suspended in the tank. At the surface of the torso were 384 electrodes, with 384 multielectrode rods that projected radially toward the center of the tank, where the canine heart was suspended in an anatomically

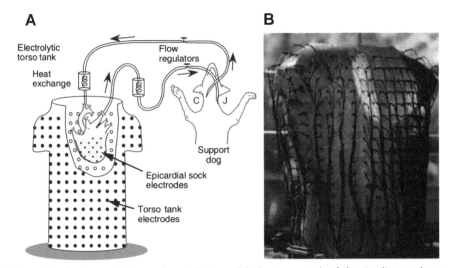

Fig. 7. (*A*) Schematic of a torso tank experimental setup. (*B*) The torso tank of the Cardiovascular and Research Training Institute, University of Utah, used to collect simultaneous epicardial and body surface potentials. ([*A*] *From* Macleod R, Brooks DH. Validation approaches for electrocardiographic inverse problems. In: Johnston P, editor. Advances in computational biomedicine, vol. 3. 3rd edition. Southampton (United Kingdom): WIT Press; 2000. p. 229–68; with permission.)

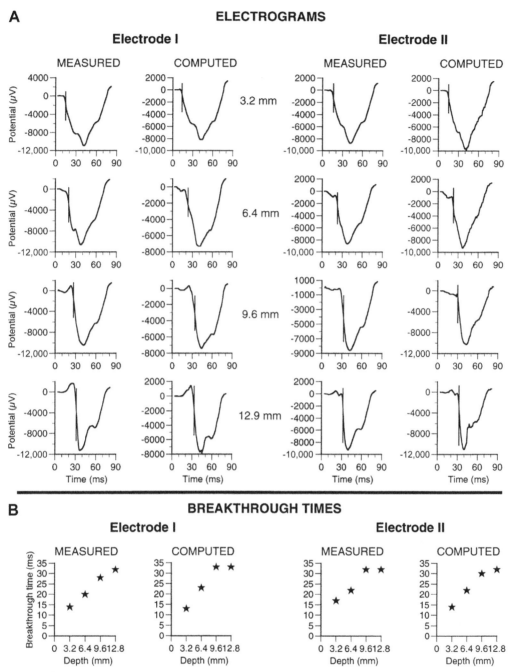

Fig. 8. Epicardial electrograms and breakthrough times. (*A*) Measured and noninvasively computed epicardial electrograms for the 2 electrode positions closest to the anterior pacing needle (electrodes I and II). Pacing depths from 3.2 to 12.9 mm relative to the epicardial surface are included. Vertical bars in the electrograms identify time of steepest negative slope (maximal −dV/dt), indicating epicardial breakthrough time. (*B*) Measured and computed breakthrough times (*stars*) versus depth of pacing. These times are correlated with the vertical bars in (*A*). Breakthrough times very similar for measured and computed values. (*From* Oster HS, Taccardi B, Lux RL, et al. Electrocardiographic imaging: noninvasive characterization of intramural myocardial activation from inverse-reconstructed epicardial potentials and electrograms. Circulation 1998;97(15):1496–507; with permission.)

correct position. In total, 918 electrodes were used within the torso. An epicardial sock of 134 electrodes provided the comparison for inverse potential reconstruction from the 384 surface leads.[59]

Noninvasively reconstructed epicardial electrograms very closely approximated those measured on the surface of the heart (**Fig. 8**). Single pacing sites could be reconstructed with a precision of 10 mm to the actual site. Despite a single minimum on the body surface potential map, dual pacing sites could be resolved with reconstructed epicardial electrograms to at least 17 mm resolution. Propagation properties such as crowded or sparse isochrones were also similar between reconstructed and measured electrograms.

A further study on a pathologic substrate was performed in a canine 4-day-old infarct model (**Fig. 9**). In this experiment, both sinus rhythm and sustained VT were studied in the torso tank setup.[65] Noninvasively obtained maps faithfully identified (1) areas of abnormal infarct substrate, (2) global activation sequences of VT, and (3) locations of epicardial breakthrough. A similar study was performed in an open chest dog model, with both forward and inverse solutions.[58]

The hybrid tank models described above afford better access to the heart and much greater flexibility of experimental design than live animal models. They have been used to evaluate inverse methods directly,[66,67] investigate the significance of inhomogeneities,[63,68] and determine the sensitivity of forward and inverse solutions to heart location,[69] pacing protocols, and various pathologic conditions.[65,70–72] Although these models can demonstrate the efficacy of different inverse algorithms, it must be kept in mind that the torso tank models are an incomplete representation of the real situation.

The target application of noninvasive imaging is the diagnosis and analysis of cardiac arrhythmias in humans, and to that end, validation in animal or human models is essential. Some of the earliest in vivo validation studies were conducted by Spach and colleagues[73] and Ramsey and colleagues[73,74] using chimpanzees and dogs, respectively. Epicardial and body surface potentials were recorded, and the corresponding electrode locations were obtained. Although the data produced from this breakthrough model have been used in other validation studies,[75] the

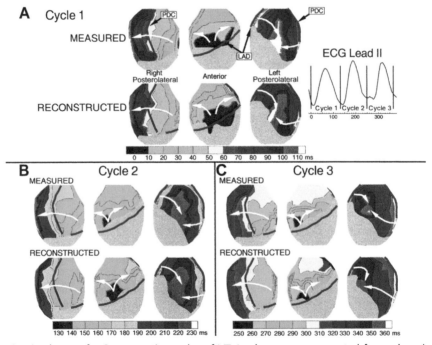

Fig. 9. Activation isochrones for 3 consecutive cycles of VT. Isochrones are presented for each cycle, with color legend (time in milliseconds) displayed below (earliest activation is *dark blue*). White arrows indicate direction of wave front propagation. Regions where no activation times are assigned are shown as gray. Electrocardiogram lead II is shown with vertical blue lines indicating the time frames displayed for each cycle. (*A*) Isochrones from VT cycle 1. Top row shows measured isochrones. Bottom row shows noninvasively reconstructed isochrones. (*B, C*) Isochrones from VT cycles 2 and 3, respectively. (*From* Burnes JE, Taccardi B, Ershler PR, et al. Noninvasive electrocardiographic imaging of substrate and intramural ventricular tachycardia in infarcted hearts. J Am Coll Cardiol 2001;38(7):2071–8; with permission.)

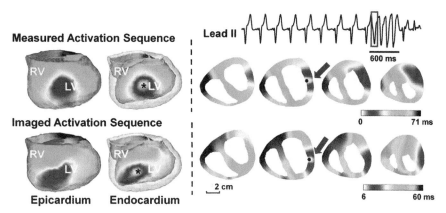

Fig. 10. A typical example of an in vivo validation study. Comparison between a measured and a reconstructed activation sequence for a nonsustained norepinephrine-induced monomorphic VT beat indicated in corresponding ECG lead II in a canine model. In the leftmost columns epicardial (*left*) and endocardial (*right*) surfaces are displayed, and horizontal sections through the heart are shown in the rightmost columns, arranged from base to apex. The pacing site and the estimated initial site of activation are marked by a black asterisk and a black spot, respectively (with a *purple arrow* in the right column). LV, left ventricle; RV, right ventricle. (*Adapted from* Han C, Pogwizd SM, Killingsworth CR, et al. Noninvasive reconstruction of the three-dimensional ventricular activation sequence during pacing and ventricular tachycardia in the canine heart. Am J Physiol Heart Circ Physiols 2012;302(1):H244–52; with permission.)

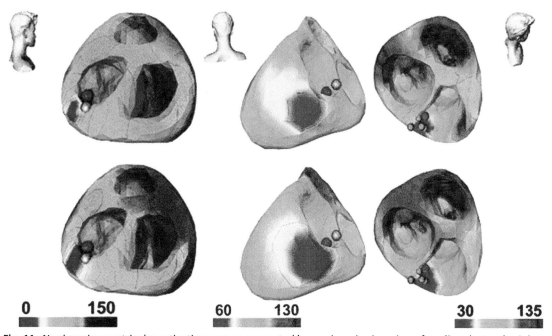

Fig. 11. Noninvasive ventricular activation map as computed by noninvasive imaging of cardiac electrophysiology in a patient with WPW syndrome. The location of earliest activation as defined by noninvasive imaging is indicated in red. The ablation points are denoted by gray markers, and the location of successful ablation is given by a purple marker, indicating the ventricular insertion site of the accessory pathway. Upper row shows activation during normal atrioventricular (AV) conduction, and lower row shows activation during adenosine-induced AV block. Head icon indicates point of view. Red and blue indicate early and late electrical activation, respectively (see color bars with activation times in milliseconds). (*Adapted from* Berger T, Fischer G, Pfeifer B, et al. Single-beat noninvasive imaging of cardiac electrophysiology of ventricular pre-excitation. J Am Coll Cardiol 2006;48(10):2045–52; with permission.)

findings have had relatively limited attention. The geometric acquisition techniques were prone to error, and models consisted of only the electrode locations. Furthermore, owing to the limited number of channels available, potentials were recorded sequentially and subsequently combined. For the next 20 years, most investigations made use of the torso tank model[64] to assess the accuracy of ECG imaging techniques. Only relatively recently have other in vivo animal models been developed. Nash and colleagues[76,77] used closed-chest anesthetized pigs to record body surface and epicardial potentials simultaneously in normal and ischemic hearts, demonstrating the repeatability of recordings between subjects, and the relationship between the pathologic condition and the resulting potential fields. Although an initial investigation of inverse model accuracy was performed,[78] a complete analysis was never reported. Simultaneous recordings of torso and transmural ventricular potentials have also been obtained in rabbits and dogs, with geometries

obtained by ultrafast CT several days before experiments.[79,80] Using these data, the accuracy of several different activation time-based inverse algorithms has been assessed in normal hearts[80,81] and during norepinephrine-induced focal VT.[25,79] More recently, this group has also used pig models.[82,83] Cardiac potentials were recorded on the endocardial surface only, whereas cardiac and torso geometries reconstructed initially using the endocardial mapping system were subsequently fused with MR images of the torso. In general, these studies demonstrate qualitative correspondence between measured and predicted activation patterns and reasonable localization of focal sources (<12 mm), a typical example of which is presented in **Fig. 10**.

Validation of inverse mapping in the clinical setting is challenging. In particular, it has not been possible to obtain simultaneous recordings of body surface potentials and cardiac potentials with high spatial resolution in closed-chest subjects. Small arrays of cardiac electrodes[84] have

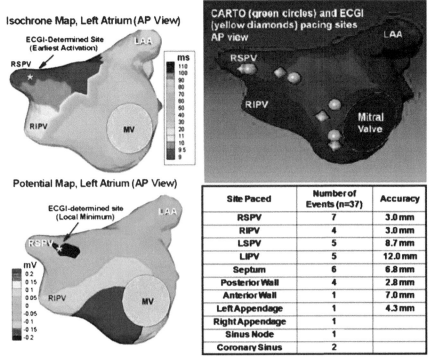

Fig. 12. ECGI accuracy locating atrial initiation sites, simulated by pacing. Top left: Isochrone map of LA (*anterior view*) with white star indicating earliest activation imaged by ECGI. Bottom left: Potential map of LA locating the minimum of earliest activation (*blue region, white star*). Top right: Merged 3D CARTO and ECGI LA images (*anterior view*). Pacing sites in RSPV, atrial septum, and anterior mitral valve annulus are shown from CARTO (*green circles*) and ECGI (*yellow diamonds*). Bottom right: Detailed information regarding pacing sites and distance between CARTO-and ECGI-imaged locations. AP, anteroposterior; LAA, left atrial appendage; MV, mitral valve; RIPV, right inferior pulmonary vein; RSPV, right superior pulmonary vein. (*From* Cuculich PS, Wang Y, Lindsay BD, et al. Noninvasive characterization of epicardial activation in humans with diverse atrial fibrillation patterns. Circulation 2010;122(14):1364–72; with permission.)

been used in the past. Alternatively, epicardial potentials recorded during open heart surgery have been combined with previously recorded body surface potentials.[54] These studies report only an approximate agreement between the reconstructed and recorded epicardial potentials with correlation coefficient between potential maps averaging approximately 0.3 over the QRS complex. Clinical validation has also been performed using endocardial surface mapping[34,53,85–87] and point-by-point epicardial mapping.[26] In the former, simulated activation sites were localized to within 15 mm of the measured locations for patients with various pathologic conditions (**Fig. 11**), but geometric inaccuracies and imprecise body surface electrode locations limited the usefulness of the epicardial mapping study. Rigorous atrial mapping compared point-by-point endocardial atrial pacing and mapping to noninvasive electrocardiographic imaging (ECGI).[88] Relative to electroanatomic maps, ECGI-determined pacing locations were accurate within 6.3 ± 3.9 mm (**Fig. 12**). Finally, several empirical studies have also been reported in which predicted epicardial activation sequences have been compared with endocardial mapping data[89,90] or a priori information.[91–93]

SUMMARY

From the dawn of the twentieth century, the ECG has revolutionized the way clinical cardiology has been practiced, and the ECG has become a cornerstone of modern medicine today. Driven by clinical and research needs for a more precise understanding of cardiac electrophysiology beyond traditional ECG, inverse solution electrocardiography has been developed, tested, and validated. Its ultimate role and acceptance as a complementary cardiac imaging modality remains to be determined, but already in its short existence, this technique is being used to help patients and drive discovery.

REFERENCES

1. Boineau JP. Electrocardiology: a 30-year perspective. J Electrocardiol 1988;21:S1–9.
2. Burdon Sanderson J, Page FJ. Experimental results relating to the rhythmical and excitatory motions of the ventricle of the frog heart. Proc Roy Soc Lond 1878;27:410–4.
3. Waller AD. A demonstration on man of electromotive changes accompanying the heart's beat. J Physiol 1887;8(5):229–34.
4. Einthoven W. Galvanometrische registratie van het menschelijk electrocardiogram. In: Herinneringsbundedl Professor S.S. Rosenstein. Leiden: Eduard Ijdo; 1902. p. 101–7.
5. Barnes AR, Pardee HE, White PD, et al. Standardization of precordial leads: supplementary report. Am Heart J 1938;15(2):235–9.
6. Wilson FN, Johnston FD, Macleod AG, et al. Electrocardiograms that represent the potential variations of a single electrode. Am Heart J 1934;9(4):447–58.
7. Goldberger E. The aVr, aVL, and aVf Leads: a simplification of standard lead electrocardiography. Am Heart J 1942;24(3):378–96.
8. Abildskov JA, Burgess MJ, Lux RL, et al. Experimental evidence for regional cardiac influence in body surface isopotential maps of dogs. Circ Res 1976;38(5):386–91.
9. Abildskov JA. Prediction of ventricular arrhythmias from ECG waveforms. J Electrocardiol 1987;20:97–101.
10. Shibata T, Kubota I, Ikeda K, et al. Body surface mapping of high-frequency components in the terminal portion during QRS complex for the prediction of ventricular tachycardia in patients with previous myocardial infarction. Circulation 1990; 82(6):2084–92.
11. Stroink G, Meeder RJ, Elliott P, et al. Arrhythmia vulnerability assessment using magnetic field maps and body surface potential maps. Pacing Clin Electrophysiol 1999;22(12):1718–28.
12. McClelland AJ, Owens CG, Menown I, et al. Comparison of the 80-lead body surface map to physician and to 12-lead electrocardiogram in detection of acute myocardial infarction. Am J Cardiol 2003; 92(3):252–7.
13. Osugi J, Ohta T, Toyama J, et al. Body surface isopotential maps in old inferior myocardial infarction undetectable by 12 lead electrocardiogram. J Electrocardiol 1984;17(1):55–62.
14. SippensGroenewegen A, Spekhorst H, Hemel NM, et al. Body surface mapping of ectopic left and right ventricular activation. QRS spectrum in patients without structural heart disease. Circulation 1990; 82(3):879–96.
15. SippensGroenewegen A, Spekhorst H, van Hemel NM, et al. Localization of the site of origin of postinfarction ventricular tachycardia by endocardial pace mapping. Body surface mapping compared with the 12-lead electrocardiogram. Circulation 1993;88(5):2290–306.
16. Guillem MS, Climent AM, Millet J, et al. Noninvasive localization of maximal frequency sites of atrial fibrillation by body surface potential mapping. Circ Arrhythm Electrophysiol 2013;6(2):294–301.
17. Ben-Haim SA, Osadchy D, Schuster I, et al. Nonfluoroscopic, in-vivo navigation and mapping technology. Nat Med 1996;2(12):1393–5.
18. Gepstein L, Hayam G, Ben-Haim SA. A novel method for nonfluoroscopic catheter-based electroanatomical mapping of the heart in-vitro and in-vivo accuracy results. Circulation 1997;95(6): 1611–22.

19. Gornick CC, Adler SW, Pederson B, et al. Validation of a new noncontact catheter system for electroanatomic mapping of left ventricular endocardium. Circulation 1999;99(6):829–35.

20. Khoury DS, Taccardi B, Lux RL, et al. Reconstruction of endocardial potentials and activation sequences from intracavitary probe measurements Localization of pacing sites and effects of myocardial structure. Circulation 1995;91(3):845–63.

21. Schilling RJ, Peters NS, Davies DW. Simultaneous endocardial mapping in the human left ventricle using a non-contact catheter: comparison of contact and reconstructed electrograms during sinus rhythm. Circulation 1998;98(9):887–98.

22. Bayley RH, Berry PM. The electrical field produced by the eccentric current dipole in the nonhomogeneous conductor. Am Heart J 1962;63(6):808–20.

23. Rudy Y, Messinger-Rapport BJ. The inverse problem in electrocardiography: solutions in terms of epicardial potentials. Crit Rev Biomed Eng 1988;16(3):215–68.

24. Cochet H, Dubois R, Sacher F, et al. Cardiac arrhythmias: multimodal assessment integrating body surface ECG mapping into cardiac imaging. Radiology 2014;271(1):239–47.

25. Han C, Pogwizd SM, Killingsworth CR, et al. Noninvasive reconstruction of the three-dimensional ventricular activation sequence during pacing and ventricular tachycardia in the canine heart. Am Heart J 2012;302(1):H244–52.

26. Sapp JL, Dawoud F, Clements JC, et al. Inverse solution mapping of epicardial potentials: quantitative comparison with epicardial contact mapping. Circ Arrhythm Electrophysiol 2012;5(5):1001–9.

27. Zhang J, Desouza KA, Cuculich PS, et al. Continuous ECGI mapping of spontaneous VT initiation, continuation, and termination with antitachycardia pacing. Heart Rhythm 2012;10(8):1244–5.

28. Rudy Y. Electrocardiographic imaging: a noninvasive imaging modality for characterization of intramural myocardial activation. J Electrocardiol 1999; 32(Suppl):1–6.

29. Rudy Y, Plonsey R, Liebman J. The effects of variations in conductivity and geometrical parameters on the electrocardiogram, utilizing eccentric spheres model. Circ Res 1979;44:104–11.

30. Rudy Y, Plonsey R. A comparison of volume conductor and source geometry effects on body surface and epicardial potentials. Circ Res 1980;46:283–91.

31. Rudy Y, Wood R, Plonsey R, et al. The effect of high lung conductivity on ECG potentials: results obtained from human subjects undergoing bronchopulmonary lavage. Circulation 1982;65:440–5.

32. Plonsey R. Bioelectric phenomena. New York: McGraw Hill; 1969.

33. Henriquez CS. Simulating the electrical behaviour of cardiac tissue using the bidomain model. Crit Rev Biomed Eng 1993;21:1–77.

34. Tilg B, Fischer G, Modre R, et al. Model-based imaging of cardiac electrical excitation in humans. IEEE Trans Med Imaging 2002;21(9):1031–9.

35. He B, Li G, Zhang X. Noninvasive three-dimensional activation time imaging of ventricular excitation by means of a heart-excitation model. Phys Med Biol 2002;47(22):4063–78.

36. Li G, He B. Localization of the site of origin of cardiac activation by means of a heart-model-based electrocardiographic imaging approach. IEEE Trans Biomed Eng 2001;48(6):660–9.

37. Colli-Franzone PC, Taccardi B, Viganotti C. An approach to inverse calculation of epicardial potentials from body surface maps. Adv Cardiol 1978;21: 50–4.

38. Barr RC, Spach MS. Inverse calculation of QRS-T epicardial potentials from body surface potential distributions for normal and ectopic beats in the intact dog. Circ Res 1978;42(5):661–75.

39. Bradley CP, Pullan AJ, Hunter PJ. Geometric modeling of the human torso using cubic hermite elements. Ann Biomed Eng 1997;25(1):96–111.

40. Pullan AJ, Bradley CP. A coupled cubic Hermite finite element/boundary element procedure for electrocardiographic problems. Comput Mech 1996; 18(5):356–68.

41. Zienkiewicz OC, Taylor RL. 4th edition. The finite element method, vol. 1. Berkshire (England): McGraw-Hill Book Company Europe; 1994. p. 150–205.

42. Wang Y, Rudy Y. Application of the method of fundamental solutions to potential-based inverse electrocardiography. Ann Biomed Eng 2006;34(8): 1272–88.

43. Martin RO, Pilkington TC. Unconstrained inverse electrocardiography: epicardial potentials. IEEE Trans Biomed Eng 1972;19(4):276–85.

44. Yamashita Y. Theoretical studies on the inverse problem in electrocardiography and the uniqueness of the solution. IEEE Trans Biomed Eng 1982;29(11): 719–25.

45. Hadamard J. Lectures on Cauchy's problems in linear partial differential equations. New Haven (CT): Yale University Press; 1923.

46. Tikhonov A, Arsenin V. Solution of ill-posed problems. Washington, DC: John Wiley & Sons; 1977.

47. Hansen PC. Rank-deficient and discrete ill-posed problems: numerical aspects of linear inversion. Philadelphia: SIAM; 1998.

48. Colli-Franzone P, Guerri L, Taccardi B, et al. Finite element approximation of regularized solutions of the inverse potential problem of electrocardiography and applications to experimental data. Calcolo 1985;22(1):91–186.

49. Golub GH, Heath MT, Wahba G. Generalized cross-validation as a method for choosing a good ridge parameter. Technometrics 1979;21(2):215–23.

50. Hansen PC, O'Leary DP. The use of the L-curve in the regularization of discrete ill-posed problems. SIAM J Sci Comput 1993;14:1487–503.

51. Johnston PR, Gulrajani RM. A new method for regularization parameter determination in the inverse problem of electrocardiography. IEEE Trans Biomed Eng 1997;44:19–32.

52. Cheng LK, Bodley JM, Pullan AJ. Comparison of potential- and activation-based formulations for the inverse problem of electrocardiology. IEEE Trans Biomed Eng 2003;50(1):11–22.

53. Modre R, Tilg B, Fischer G, et al. Atrial noninvasive activation mapping of paced rhythm data. J Cardiovasc Electrophysiol 2003;14(7):712–9.

54. Shahidi AV, Savard P, Nadeau R. Forward and inverse problems of electrocardiography: modeling and recovery of epicardial potentials in humans. IEEE Trans Biomed Eng 1994;41(3):249–56.

55. Calvetti D, Reichel L, Sgallari F, et al. An iterative method for image reconstruction from projections. In: Lewis JG, editor. Proceedings of the Fifth SIAM Conference on Applied Linear Algebra. Philadelphia: SIAM; 1994. p. 92–6.

56. Ramanathan C, Jia P, Ghanem R, et al. Noninvasive electrocardiographic imaging (ECGI): application of the generalized minimal residual (GMRes) method. Ann Biomed Eng 2003;31(8):981–94.

57. Saad Y, Schultz MH. GMRes: a generalized minimal residual algorithm for solving nonsymmetric linear systems. SIAM J Sci Stat Comput 1986;7:856–69.

58. Burnes JE, Taccardi B, MacLeod RS, et al. Noninvasive ECG imaging of electrophysiologically abnormal substrates in infarcted hearts: a model study. Circulation 2000;101(5):533–40.

59. Oster HS, Taccardi B, Lux RL, et al. Electrocardiographic imaging: noninvasive characterization of intramural myocardial activation from inverse-reconstructed epicardial potentials and electrograms. Circulation 1998;97(15):1496–507.

60. Buist ML, Smith NP, Pullan AJ. Cardiac electromechanics and the forward/inverse problems of electrocardiology. Proceedings of the Annual International IEEE EMBS Conference. Shanghai (China); 2005. p. 7198–200.

61. Klepfer RN, Johnson CR, MacLeod RS. The effects of inhomogeneities and anisotropies on electrocardiographic fields: a 3-D finite-element study. IEEE Trans Biomed Eng 1997;44(8):706–19.

62. Messinger-Rapport BJ, Rudy Y. Noninvasive recovery of epicardial potentials in a realistic heart-torso geometry. Normal sinus rhythm. Circ Res 1990;66(4):1023–39.

63. Burger HC, Van Milaan JB. Heart-vector and leads: part II. Heart 1947;9(3):154–60.

64. Nagata Y. The influence of the inhomogeneities of electrical conductivity within the torso on the electrocardiogram as evaluated from the view point of the transfer impedance vector. Jpn Heart J 1970;11(5):489–505.

65. Burnes JE, Taccardi B, Ershler PR, et al. Noninvasive electrocardiographic imaging of substrate and intramural ventricular tachycardia in infarcted hearts. J Am Coll Cardiol 2001;38(7):2071–8.

66. Oster HS, Taccardi B, Lux RL, et al. Electrocardiographic imaging: evaluating its ability to locate and resolve pacing sites noninvasively. In: Proc. Ann. Int. IEEE EMBS. Baltimore (MD): IEEE; 1994. p. 151–2.

67. Rudy Y, Taccardi B. Noninvasive imaging and catheter imaging of potentials, electrograms, and isochrones on the ventricular surfaces. J Electrocardiol 1997;30(Suppl):19–23.

68. Grayzel J, Lizzi F. The combined influence of inhomogeneities and dipole location. Bipolar ECG leads in the frontal plane. Am Heart J 1967;74(4):503–12.

69. MacLeod RS, Ni Q, Punske B, et al. Effects of heart position on the body-surface electrocardiogram. J Electrocardiol 2000;33(Suppl):229–37.

70. Lux RL, Fuller MS, MacLeod RS, et al. Noninvasive indices of repolarization and its dispersion. J Electrocardiol 1999;32(Suppl):153–7.

71. MacLeod RS, Taccardi B, Lux RL. Electrocardiographic mapping in a realistic torso tank preparation. In: Proc. Ann. Int. IEEE EMBS. Montreal (Canada): IEEE; 1995. p. 245–6.

72. MacLeod RS, Punske B, Yilmaz B, et al. The role of heart rate in myocardial ischemia from restricted coronary perfusion. J Electrocardiol 2001; 34(Suppl):43–51.

73. Spach MS, Barr RC, Lanning CF, et al. Origin of body surface QRS and T wave potentials from epicardial potential distributions in the intact chimpanzee. Circulation 1977;55(2):268.

74. Ramsey M, Barr RC, Spach MS. Comparison of measured torso potentials with those simulated from epicardial potentials for ventricular depolarization and repolarization in the intact dog. Circ Res 1977;41(5):660–72.

75. Stanley PC, Pilkington TC, Morrow MN. The effects of thoracic inhomogeneities on the relationship between epicardial and torso potentials. IEEE Trans Biomed Eng 1986;33(3):273–84. http://dx.doi.org/10.1109/TBME.1986.325711.

76. Nash MP, Bradley CP, Cheng LK, et al. An experimental-computational framework for validating in-vivo ECG inverse algorithms. Int J Bioelectromagn 2000;2(2):1–7.

77. Nash MP, Bradley CP, Paterson DJ. Imaging electrocardiographic dispersion of depolarization and repolarization during ischemia: simultaneous body surface and epicardial mapping. Circulation 2003; 107(17):2257–63.

78. Nash MP, Bradley CP, Cheng LK, et al. Electrocardiographic inverse validation study: in-vivo mapping and analysis. FASEB J 2000;14(4):A442.

79. Han C, Pogwizd SM, Killingsworth CR, et al. Noninvasive three-dimensional cardiac activation imaging

of ventricular arrhythmias in the rabbit heart. Comput Cardiol 2010;37:125–7.

80. Zhang X, Ramachandra I, Liu Z, et al. Three-dimensional activation sequence reconstruction from body surface potential maps by means of a heart-model-based imaging approach. In: Comput. Cardiol. (vol. 31). Chicago (IL): IEEE; 2004. p. 1–4.

81. Han C, Liu Z, Zhang X, et al. Noninvasive three-dimensional cardiac activation imaging from body surface potential maps: a computational and experimental study on a rabbit model. IEEE Trans Med Imaging 2008;27(11):1622–30.

82. Liu C, Skadsberg ND, Ahlberg SE, et al. Estimation of global ventricular activation sequences by noninvasive three-dimensional electrical imaging: validation studies in a Swine model during pacing. J Cardiovasc Electrophysiol 2008;19(5):535–40.

83. Liu C, Iaizzo PA, He B. Three-dimensional imaging of ventricular activation and electrograms from intracavitary recordings. IEEE Trans Biomed Eng 2011; 58(4):868–75.

84. Ghanem RN, Jia P, Ramanathan C, et al. Noninvasive electrocardiographic imaging (ECGI): comparison to intraoperative mapping in patients. Heart Rhythm 2005;2(4):339–54.

85. Berger T, Fischer G, Pfeifer B, et al. Single-beat noninvasive imaging of cardiac electrophysiology of ventricular pre-excitation. J Am Coll Cardiol 2006;48(10):2045–52.

86. Fischer G, Hanser F, Pfeifer B, et al. A signal processing pipeline for noninvasive imaging of ventricular preexcitation. Methods Inf Med 2005; 44(4):508–15.

87. Modre R, Tilg B, Fischer G, et al. Ventricular surface activation time imaging from electrocardiogram mapping data. Med Biol Eng Comput 2004;42(2): 146–50.

88. Cuculich PS, Wang Y, Lindsay BD, et al. Noninvasive characterization of epicardial activation in humans with diverse atrial fibrillation patterns. Circulation 2010;122(14):1364–72.

89. MacLeod RS, Miller R, Gardner MJ, et al. Application of an electrocardiographic inverse solution to localize myocardial ischemia during percutaneous transluminal coronary angioplasty. J Cardiovasc Electrophysiol 1995;6(1):2–18.

90. Wang Y, Cuculich PS, Zhang J, et al. Noninvasive electroanatomic mapping of human ventricular arrhythmias with electrocardiographic imaging. Sci Transl Med 2011;3(98):98ra84.

91. Cheng LK, Buist ML, Sands GB, et al. Interpretation of ECG signals through forward and inverse modelling. In: Proc. Ann. Int. IEEE EMBS (vol. 2). Houston (TX): IEEE; 2002. p. 1389–90.

92. Ramanathan C, Ghanem RN, Jia P, et al. Noninvasive electrocardiographic imaging for cardiac electrophysiology and arrhythmia. Nat Med 2004;10(4): 422–8.

93. Ramanathan C, Jia P, Ghanem RN, et al. Activation and repolarization of the normal human heart under complete physiological conditions. Proc Natl Acad Sci U S A 2006;103(16):6309–14.

Electrocardiographic Imaging of Heart Rhythm Disorders: From Bench to Bedside

Yoram Rudy, PhD[a],*, Bruce D. Lindsay, MD[b]

KEYWORDS

- Electrocardiographic imaging • Cardiac resynchronization • Ventricular tachycardia
- Atrial tachycardia • Atrial fibrillation

KEY POINTS

- Noninvasive electrocardiographic imaging (ECGI; also called ECG mapping) can reconstruct potentials, electrograms, activation sequences, and repolarization patterns on the epicardial surface of the heart with high resolution.
- ECGI maps show normal right ventricular activation and diverse patterns of delayed left ventricular activation in patients with heart failure.
- ECGI can possibly be used to quantify synchrony, identify potential responders/nonresponders to cardiac resynchronization therapy, and guide electrode placement for effective resynchronization therapy.
- ECGI accurately determines the origins of focal atrial and ventricular arrhythmias; it also accurately defines atrial and ventricular macro-reentrant circuits.
- ECGI recordings of atrial fibrillation highlight differences in the complexity of atrial activation in patients with paroxysmal compared with persistent atrial fibrillation.
- Multiple wavelets are observed in a high percentage of patients with atrial fibrillation, and focal mechanisms can be demonstrated in pulmonary and nonpulmonary vein origins.
- During atrial fibrillation, wave fronts vary continuously over time and space; repetitive wave-front patterns and focal drivers provide potential targets for ablation of atrial fibrillation.

INTRODUCTION

Noninvasive evaluation of the electrical status of the heart and noninvasive diagnosis of cardiac arrhythmias are still based on the standard electrocardiogram (ECG), which records signals on the body surface, far away from the heart. The ECG has been a most useful clinical tool for more than 100 years. However, because it records the reflection of cardiac excitation as seen far from the heart at a limited number of sites, it lacks sensitivity and specificity, and its spatial resolution is very low. Moreover, each individual ECG electrode records

Funding Sources: NIH-NHLBI grants R01-HL-033343 and R01-HL-049054 (to Y. Rudy) and Washington University Institute of Clinical and Translational Sciences grant UL1 TR000448 from the National Center for Advancing Translational Sciences (NCATS) of the NIH. Y. Rudy is the Fred Saigh Distinguished Professor at Washington University.

Disclosures: Dr Y. Rudy co-chairs the scientific advisory board, holds equity in, and receives royalties from CardioInsight Technologies (CIT). CIT does not support any research conducted in Dr Y. Rudy's laboratory.

[a] Cardiac Bioelectricity and Arrhythmia Center, Washington University, Campus Box 1097, St Louis, MO 63130-4899, USA; [b] Clinical Cardiac Electrophysiology, Cardiovascular Medicine, Cleveland Clinic Foundation, 9500 Euclid Avenue/J2-2, Cleveland, OH 44195, USA

* Corresponding author.

E-mail address: rudy@wustl.edu

Card Electrophysiol Clin 7 (2015) 17–35

http://dx.doi.org/10.1016/j.ccep.2014.11.013

the integrated signal generated by activity over the entire heart.[1,2] Consequently, geometric information on cardiac location of electrophysiologic events (eg, a focus of focal arrhythmia, or the circuit of a reentrant arrhythmia) is lost in the ECG. To overcome these limitations, invasive mapping techniques, using intracardiac catheters, have been developed and used extensively for diagnosis and guidance of therapy. Many arrhythmias require that mapping be conducted simultaneously over the atria or ventricles with sufficient spatial resolution, and continuously in time over a sufficiently long duration. These requirements cannot be met with current invasive, catheter-based mapping techniques. Moreover, the risk, complexity, and cost of invasive mapping limit its application for arrhythmic risk stratification and repeated follow-up tests following therapy. Clearly a method for noninvasive mapping of the heart's electrical activity is much desired; it would serve cardiac electrophysiology in a similar role to that of established noninvasive imaging modalities (computed tomography [CT], MRI, and ultrasonography) used extensively in the practice of modern medicine.

Motivated by this need, Electrocardiographic imaging (ECGI) was developed in Rudy's laboratory for application in cardiac patients.[3] ECGI (also called electrocardiographic mapping [ECM]) reconstructs potentials, electrograms, activation sequences (isochrones), and repolarization patterns on the heart surface. The reconstruction is performed simultaneously over the entire heart and is done continuously on a beat-by-beat basis. This article provides a brief description of the ECGI procedure and selected previously published examples of its application in important clinical conditions, including heart failure (HF) and cardiac resynchronization therapy (CRT),[4–6] atrial arrhythmias,[7–9] and ventricular tachycardia (VT).[10] All reported studies were approved by the Institutional Review Board of the participating institutions (University Hospitals of Cleveland, the Cleveland Clinic and Washington University in St Louis), and informed consent was obtained from all patients.

THE ELECTROCARDIOGRAPHIC IMAGING METHOD

ECGI computes potentials on the epicardial surface of the heart from recorded body surface potentials, a procedure that solves the inverse problem of electrocardiography, formulated in terms of potentials[2,11,12] (the forward problem computes body surface potentials from epicardial potentials). In mathematical terms, this constitutes an inverse solution to Laplace's equation, which describes the electric potential field in the volume between the heart surface and the body surface. The inverse problem is ill posed, meaning that even small errors in the measured data (measurement noise, uncertainty in electrode positions) can result in very large errors in the computed epicardial potentials. To suppress these errors, the authors have applied 2 different computational schemes in the ECGI application: Tikhonov regularization[13] (a method that imposes constraints on the solution) and the generalized minimal residual (GMRes) iterative technique.[14] From the time sequence of computed epicardial potentials, ECGI constructs electrograms (EGMs) at many locations on the epicardium and, from these, the epicardial activation sequence (isochrones) and repolarization pattern.

In addition to the electrocardiographic potential over the entire torso surface, the ECGI algorithm requires knowledge of the geometries of the heart and torso surfaces. To obtain the torso potentials, 250 electrodes mounted on strips or in a vest are applied to the patient's torso (both anterior and posterior) and connected to a mapping system (**Fig. 1**). The electrodes are sampled at 1-millisecond intervals. Each electrode contains a marker that is visible on a CT scan. The patient undergoes thoracic noncontrast gated CT scanning with axial resolution of 3 mm, providing the epicardial geometry and torso electrode positions in the same frame of reference. The recorded torso potential and CT-derived geometric information provide the input data for the ECGI algorithm. The computation of epicardial potentials, EGMs, and activation/repolarization sequences is performed during a single beat and does not require the accumulation of data from many beats. This property makes it possible to image nonsustained and polymorphic arrhythmias, and arrhythmias that are not hemodynamically tolerated. It is noteworthy that the authors use very low radiation during the CT scan (less than 2 rad), and this is further decreasing with improving CT technology. For longitudinal studies over time, only one CT scan is obtained at the first ECGI procedure. The authors have used MRI instead of CT in subjects without implanted devices; once it becomes safe to apply MRI in the presence of such devices, the use of MRI could be expanded. It is also conceivable that in the future high-quality 3-dimensional echocardiography could be used to obtain the geometry.

ECGI has been validated extensively under different physiologic and pathologic conditions in animal models, including a human-shaped torso-tank with a perfused dog heart suspended

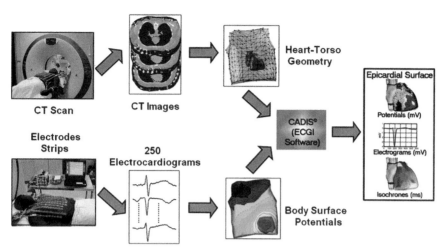

Fig. 1. The electrocardiographic imaging (ECGI) procedure. (*Bottom*) Recording the body surface electrical data with 250 electrodes. (*Top*) Obtaining the geometric data using computed tomography (CT). The ECGI software algorithms combine the electrical and geometric data to produce maps of potentials, electrograms, activation, and repolarization on the epicardial surface of the heart. (*Adapted from* Ramanathan C, Ghanem RN, Jia P, et al. Noninvasive electrocardiographic imaging for cardiac electrophysiology and arrhythmia. Nat Med 2004;10:423; with permission.)

in the correct anatomic position.[15–19] In this setup, torso potentials (the ECGI input) were measured simultaneously with epicardial potentials that provided a gold standard for evaluating the accuracy of ECGI. Experiments were conducted in normal and infarcted hearts during sinus rhythm, multiple-site pacing, and reentrant VT. Correlation coefficients between ECGI generated and directly measured epicardial EGMs were greater than 0.9 for 72% of all epicardial locations, indicating very good agreement. Validation in humans included comparison with direct intraoperative mapping in patients undergoing open heart surgery during sinus rhythm and right ventricular (RV) epicardial and endocardial pacing (**Fig. 2**).[20]

It must be emphasized that ECGI is not body surface potential mapping (BSPM), as there is confusion in the literature regarding the difference between these two terms that are sometimes used interchangeably. BSPM is only an extension of the body surface ECG, accomplished through the application of a large number of electrodes to the torso surface. The output of BSPM is potentials on the body surface, not on the heart. By contrast, ECGI provides cardiac electrophysiologic data on the heart, and maps cardiac electrical excitation in relation to the heart's anatomy.

THE ELECTROPHYSIOLOGIC SUBSTRATE OF HEART FAILURE

Delayed ventricular activation, predominantly of the left ventricle, accompanies more than 30% of

moderate to severe HF cases.[21] Body surface electrocardiographic characteristics in many HF patients include a wide QRS complex and a left bundle branch block (LBBB) pattern[22]; this provides some insight on the global excitation sequence. However, a detailed description of activation patterns in the in situ heart of HF patients has been lacking. Taking advantage of its noninvasive nature, the authors used ECGI to obtain this information. The patient population included 8 HF patients (6 men, 2 women; age 72 ± 11 years; New York Heart Association functional class III–IV) with ventricular conduction delay, receiving CRT through an implanted atrial-biventricular (BiV) pacing device.[4]

Fig. 3 shows the epicardial activation sequences (isochrone maps) during native rhythm (NR) in 4 HF patients (4 top rows). The bottom row shows an isochrone map of a normal heart for reference. In all HF patients, activation of the right ventricle is completely normal. RV epicardial excitation starts from a breakthrough site (round isochrone) at the typical normal location, indicating a normally functioning right bundle of the specialized conduction system. As in normal hearts,[23,24] there is radial, uniform spread of excitation from the breakthrough site, with the basal or anterior/inferior paraseptal regions activating last. Areas of conduction slowing (indicated by crowding of isochrones) or conduction block (thick black lines) are not present in the right ventricle. Mean duration of RV activation was 25 milliseconds, similar to normal.

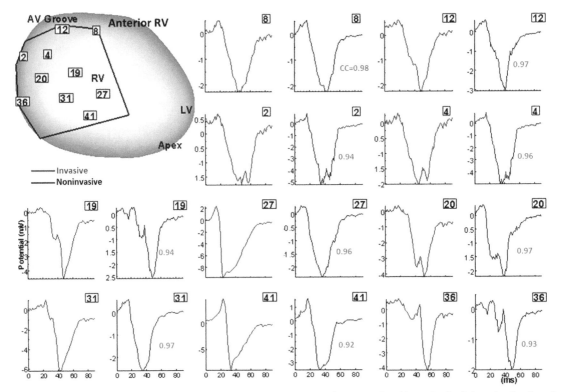

Fig. 2. Validation of ECGI in patients undergoing intraoperative cardiac mapping (sinus rhythm). Invasive (*red*) and noninvasive ECGI reconstructed (*black*) QRS epicardial electrograms from corresponding positions on anterior RV (framed numbers) are shown side by side. Correlation coefficients (CC) are provided for each pair. The intraoperative recording patch boundaries and electrode positions are marked on the heart image. Similar results were obtained for posterior LV. AV, atrioventricular; LV, left ventricle; RV, right ventricle. (*From* Ghanem RN, Jia P, Ramanathan C, et al. Noninvasive electrocardiographic imaging (ECGI): comparison to intraoperative mapping in patients. Heart Rhythm 2005;2:344; with permission.)

By contrast, left ventricular (LV) activation is delayed in all patients, accounting for the LBBB pattern of the body surface ECG. Unlike RV activation, which is similar for all patients, LV activation patterns are heterogeneous and different among patients, with variable locations of lines of conduction block (thick black lines) and regions of slow conduction (crowded isochrones). Of importance, the location of latest activation (blue) varies greatly. A common occurrence is the presence of anterior lines of block, which prevent the activation front from propagating deeper into the left ventricle after crossing the interventricular septum from the right ventricle; the wave front propagates in a U-shaped pattern to reach the lateral wall by way of the apical or inferior left ventricle. This U-shaped pattern was also observed with invasive catheter mapping.[25] As a consequence of the delayed and regionally nonuniform excitation, ventricular activation becomes desynchronized, leading to reduced cardiac function.

Cardiac Resynchronization Therapy

CRT applies BiV pacing to restore ventricular synchrony. Through pacing, it attempts to accelerate excitation of the most delayed LV activation region. CRT has been shown to improve patients' symptoms, LV performance, and long-term survival in approximately 70% of cases (~33% of patients do not respond to CRT).[26] The ability to achieve synchrony with CRT depends on the site of LV lead placement. As seen in the ECGI maps of **Fig. 3**, the region of most delayed LV activation (the desired pacing location) is variable and patient specific (compare the dark blue regions in patients #7 and #3). Also, other properties of the electrophysiologic substrate should be taken into consideration when deciding on lead placement.

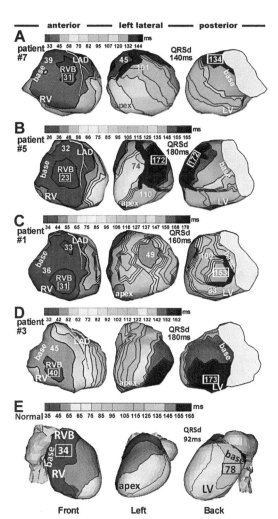

Fig. 3. Epicardial activation maps of native rhythm (NR) in 4 representative patients with heart failure (HF) (A–D) and in a normal heart (E). Three views are shown for each heart, as indicated at the bottom. Thick black lines indicate conduction block. All HF maps show sequential activation of right ventricle (RV) followed by greatly delayed activation of left ventricle (LV) (left bundle branch block [LBBB] pattern). RV activation is normal in all patients. LV activation patterns vary among patients; importantly, there is wide variation in the region of latest LV activation. Normal activation (E) is highly synchronized, without conduction delays or block. Numbers indicate activation times (from QRS onset) in milliseconds. Earliest and latest ventricular activation times are indicated by framed numbers. LAD, left anterior descending coronary artery; QRSd, QRS duration; RVB, right ventricular epicardial breakthrough. (Adapted from Jia P, Ramanathan C, Ghanem RN, et al. Electrocardiographic imaging of cardiac resynchronization therapy in heart failure: observations of variable electrophysiologic responses. Heart Rhythm 2006;3:300; with permission.)

For example, in patient #1 the region of latest activation (blue; 153 milliseconds) is surrounded by a line of block and slow conduction, and pacing from this region is unlikely to capture. Mapping of the substrate with ECGI before CRT device implantation can provide useful information for guiding optimal electrode placement. **Fig. 4** shows an example of ECGI-guided electrode placement in the area of latest activation in a pediatric HF patient with congenital heart disease.[5]

Responders to Cardiac Resynchronization Therapy

Fig. 5 shows epicardial activation during both NR (top row of each panel) and BiV pacing (bottom row of each panel) in 2 patients (Panel A, #5; Panel B, #3). The LV pacing lead of patient #5 was located at the lateral wall (see **Fig. 5**A, white asterisk). Activation from the pacing site captured most of the left ventricle and eliminated the very late activation region at 174 milliseconds during NR. The line of block on the anterior left ventricle, present during NR, was maintained during BiV, although its geometry was somewhat modified. Latest activation occurred at the anterior left ventricle, adjacent to this line of block, at 138 milliseconds. Relative to NR, ventricular activation was much better synchronized during BiV. Patient #3 (see **Fig. 5**B) had an anterior LV lead, which captured the left ventricle and eliminated the very late activation region at 173 milliseconds, present during NR. A functional line of block, not present during NR, emerged anterolaterally during BiV pacing. LV activation pivoted around this block and ended at lateral basal left ventricle at 117 milliseconds, with much better electrical synchrony than during NR. Both patients responded well to CRT as judged by postimplant echo parameters.

Nonresponders to Cardiac Resynchronization Therapy

Fig. 6 shows examples of patients who did not respond to CRT. Patient #8 had a lateral LV lead (see **Fig. 6**A). While pacing from this site captured the late LV basal region, activated at 120 milliseconds during NR, it created an anterolateral functional line of block that forced the wave front to pivot and activate a large portion of anterior left ventricle very late and asynchronously at 132 milliseconds. **Fig. 6**B shows patient #4 who had an anterior LV pacing lead. LV lateral wall activation was slowed relative to NR and took twice as long to reach the basal left ventricle (dark blue, at 187 milliseconds).

Pre- and Post-CRT Activation-Isochrones in Patient #6

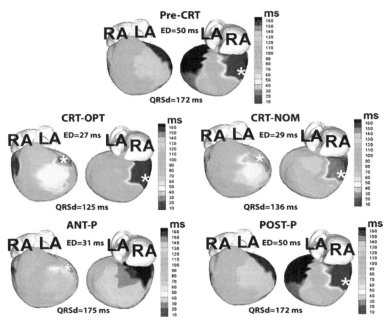

Fig. 4. Guidance of lead placement with ECGI. Activation maps for 5 pacing regimes (Pre-CRT, CRT-OPT, CRT-NOM, ANT-P, POST-P) are shown in 2 views, anterior (*left*) and inferior (*right*). This patient is an 8-year-old male with hypoplastic left heart syndrome, mitral atresia, and double-outlet right ventricle who had a DDD epicardial pacemaker implanted at the age of 3 months for postoperative complete heart block. The pacing lead was placed in a right posterior area (*white asterisk*, pre-CRT panel). At 4 years of age, he had a fenestrated extracardiac Fontan operation. Over the following several years he developed worsening HF. His pre-CRT activation map (*top panel*) showed a severely elevated electrical dyssynchrony (ED) index (ED = 50 milliseconds; see text for definition of ED), with severely delayed activation of the left anterior basal and inferior basal areas of the ventricle (*dark blue*, pre-CRT). These areas were designated as suitable sites for the resynchronization lead. The patient underwent surgical implant of an epicardial lead at the left anterior basal area. Repeated ECGI 3 months after implant showed a dramatically improved synchrony during optimal biventricular (BiV) pacing, with ED dropping to the normal range (ED = 27 milliseconds; CRT-OPT); improvement with nominal BiV pacing (without optimization of interventricular pacing delay) was slightly less (ED = 29 milliseconds; CRT-NOM). ANT-P, anterior lead pacing only; CRT, cardiac resynchronization therapy; LA, left atrium; POST-P, posterior lead pacing only; RA, right atrium. White asterisks denote sites of pacing leads. (*From* Silva JN, Ghosh S, Bowman TM, et al. Cardiac resynchronization therapy in pediatric congenital heart disease: insights from noninvasive electrocardiographic imaging. Heart Rhythm 2009;6:1183; with permission.)

It must be noted that the electrophysiologic substrate is dynamic; it depends on the activation pattern, and changes in response to pacing. With changing direction and orientation of the activation fronts relative to the anatomic structure of the myocardium, new functional lines of block and regions of slow conduction emerge while others disappear. ECGI can capture these dynamic changes because it maps the activation continuously with a panoramic view of the ventricles. ECGI has also been able to delineate the electrophysiologic substrate associated with postmyocardial infarction scars.[27,28]

The ECGI observation that RV activation is normal in HF and utilizes the specialized conduction system suggested that CRT can be achieved with LV pacing alone. The authors demonstrated in 3 of 4 patients with atrioventricular conduction that with optimal atrioventricular delay, synchronization was achieved by fusion between intrinsic excitation from the RV electrode and paced excitation from the LV electrode (see Figure 7 in Ref.[4]).

Evaluating and Quantifying Synchrony with Electrocardiographic Imaging

As mentioned earlier, each ECG electrode on the body surface records a signal that is generated by activity in the entire heart. Consequently, a fundamental limitation of the body surface ECG is its inability to provide accurate information about regional activation in the heart and the spatial-temporal relationships between activities in different regions. By definition, this relationship is precisely what determines the degree of electrical synchrony. Despite this limitation, the QRS duration (QRSd) on the body surface ECG has been used as an index of cardiac electrical synchrony, with the interpretation that a longer

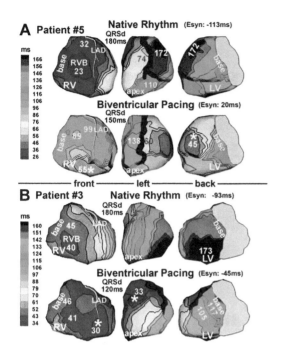

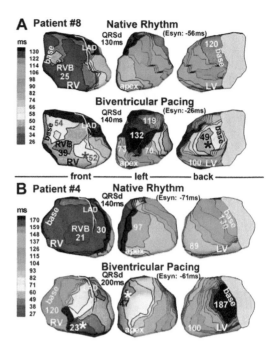

Fig. 5. (*A, B*) Activation maps from 2 patients who responded to CRT. NR (*top*) and BiV pacing (*bottom*) maps are shown for each patient. The format is similar to that in **Fig. 3**. Pacing sites are marked by asterisks. (*From* Jia P, Ramanathan C, Ghanem RN, et al. Electrocardiographic imaging of cardiac resynchronization therapy in heart failure: observations of variable electrophysiologic responses. Heart Rhythm 2006;3:302; with permission.)

Fig. 6. (*A, B*) Activation maps from 2 patients who did not respond to CRT. NR (*top*) and BiV pacing (*bottom*) maps are shown for each patient. The format is similar to that in **Fig. 3**. Pacing sites are marked by asterisks. (*From* Jia P, Ramanathan C, Ghanem RN, et al. Electrocardiographic imaging of cardiac resynchronization therapy in heart failure: observations of variable electrophysiologic responses. Heart Rhythm 2006;3:303; with permission.)

QRSd indicates reduced synchrony.[29] The QRSd is noninvasive and easily obtainable; however, it is only an estimate of the duration of global ventricular activation as reflected on the body surface ECG. As an illustration of its limitation in measuring synchrony, a small region of delayed activation that is insignificant to overall synchrony and cardiac function can skew the QRSd to very long values. In contrast to the body surface ECG, ECGI reconstructs the pattern of regional electrical activity in the heart and the spatial-temporal relationships between activities in the different regions, which define the degree of synchrony. Using ECGI activation maps, the authors defined and computed an intra-LV electrical dyssynchrony (ED) index as the standard deviation of activation times at 500 sites on the LV epicardium, including the epicardial aspect of the septum.[6] ED, by definition, is a measure of the spatial dispersion of activation times across the left ventricle, and depends on how much of the left ventricle activates late relative to the rest of LV myocardium. The control value of ED in a population of 22 young

healthy subjects without HF was determined at 20 ± 4 milliseconds; the left ventricle is defined to be electrically asynchronous when ED is 28 milliseconds or greater.

Fig. 7 illustrates the usefulness of ED as an index of electrical synchrony. It shows ECGI activation maps of a patient who responded to CRT. Although his native QRSd is normal at only 100 milliseconds, the native activation pattern (NAT) (see **Fig. 7**) is very dyssynchronous (ED = 32 milliseconds), characterized by lines of block and delayed activation of extensive areas of the LV lateral and inferior wall (blue in the NAT panel of **Fig. 7**). CRT restores LV synchrony and reduces ED to a normal value of 20 milliseconds.

In an ECGI study of 25 HF patients undergoing CRT,[6] the authors observed that LV electrical dyssynchrony is consistently high (ED ~30 milliseconds) for native QRSd greater than 130 milliseconds. However, among patients with native QRSd of approximately 130 milliseconds, ED varied widely. Four patients with QRSd between 120 and 130 milliseconds had synchronized LV activation (ED <28 milliseconds); as could have

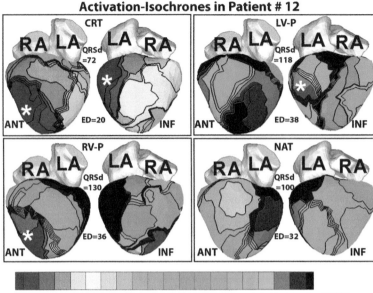

Activation-Isochrones in Patient # 12

15 19 23 27 31 35 39 43 47 51 55 59 63 67 71 75 79 83 87 **ms**

Fig. 7. Activation maps in a patient who had a normal QRSd despite LBBB pattern before implant. Note the large electrical dyssynchrony (ED = 32 milliseconds) in the native rhythm (*NAT panel*) despite a normal QRS duration (QRSd = 100 milliseconds). Cardiac resynchronization therapy (*CRT panel*) restored electrical synchrony (ED = 20 milliseconds) in the normal range. Pacing sites are indicated by asterisks. Each panel shows anterior (ANT, *left*) and inferior (INF, *right*) 4-chamber views. RV-P and LV-P indicate RV pacing only or LV pacing only, respectively. (*From* Ghosh S, Silva JN, Canham RM, et al. Electrophysiologic substrate and intraventricular left ventricular dyssynchrony in nonischemic heart failure patients undergoing cardiac resynchronization therapy. Heart Rhythm 2011;8:697; with permission.)

been predicted, all of them were nonresponders to CRT because their left ventricle was already synchronized in NR. Two patients had very dyssynchronous LV activation (ED = 32 and 34 milliseconds) during NR despite QRSd less than 120 milliseconds; they both responded to CRT. These data suggest that the ECGI-determined ED could complement the QRSd as a predictor of CRT response, especially in the range of QRSd between 100 and 130 milliseconds whereby QRSd is not a reliable index of synchrony. This result is illustrated further in the scatter plots of **Fig. 8**, which show only very weak correlation between ED and QRSd. During NR (NAT), for the range of QRSd less than 130 milliseconds, ED is a sensitive index of synchrony but QRSd shows little variation between patients (red elliptical frame).

VENTRICULAR ARRHYTHMIAS

Symptomatic ventricular arrhythmias often are not responsive to medical therapy, or the medications required to suppress the arrhythmia are not tolerated. Ablation of ventricular arrhythmias has evolved to become a major treatment option for patients with symptomatic premature ventricular contractions (PVCs) or sustained ventricular arrhythmias. The major challenges of ablation therapy are that the arrhythmia may not occur

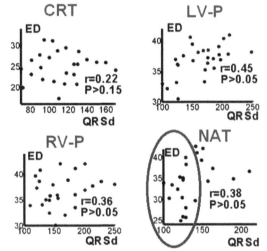

Fig. 8. Scatter plots of electrical dyssynchrony (ED) versus QRSd for CRT rhythm; left ventricular paced rhythm (LV-P); right ventricular paced rhythm (RV-P); and native sinus rhythm (NAT). r is the Pearson correlation coefficient; *P*<.05 is considered a significant correlation. The red elliptical frame indicates the NR (NAT) for the range of QRSd less than 130 milliseconds during NR (NAT). (*From* Ghosh S, Silva JN, Canham RM, et al. Electrophysiologic substrate and intraventricular left ventricular dyssynchrony in nonischemic heart failure patients undergoing cardiac resynchronization therapy. Heart Rhythm 2011;8:698; with permission.)

spontaneously or be inducible at the time of study, and in some patients the hemodynamic instability of VT poses an important limitation on accurate identification of the mechanism and site of origin of the arrhythmia. Moreover, point-by-point mapping with an ablation catheter may not provide sufficient detail to determine the origin, and patients often have multiple VT morphologies representing different circuits that increase the difficulty of the procedure and may compromise the long-term outcome.

Simultaneous acquisition of global ventricular activation offers promise for rapid and accurate identification of the mechanism of VT that could guide ablation of the critical elements, expedite the time required to perform the procedure, and improve outcomes of arrhythmias that are difficult to map using standard point-by-point endocardial mapping.

Preliminary studies have shown that ECGI accurately identifies the site of early ventricular activation in patients with accessory pathways,[30,31] distinguishes the origin of premature ventricular contractions,[10,32,33] and can be used to construct the activation sequence of reentrant VT.[10] **Fig. 9** shows examples of epicardial activation recorded

using ECGI in 4 patients with focal mechanisms arising from the RV outflow tract (RVOT) and different sites within left ventricles that were concordant with endocardial mapping. **Fig. 10** demonstrates epicardial ventricular activation during a sinus capture beat compared with reentrant VT with early activation of a region on the border of a scar documented by nuclear imaging. In some patients, adjacent but anatomically distinct origins, such as the RVOT and coronary cusps, may take time to differentiate using standard catheter-based point-by-point mapping. **Fig. 11** was recorded from an ECGI prototype developed for commercial use by CardioInsight (Cleveland, OH, USA). It correctly identifies the origin of a premature ventricular contraction arising from the left coronary cusp.

Fig. 12 provides an example of reentry on the lateral wall of the left ventricle in a patient with an infiltrative cardiomyopathy. Although there is some beat-to-beat variation in activation that would not be appreciated with point-by-point mapping, the wave front of activation propagated to the LV lateral base where it reached a line of block in the inferolateral base.

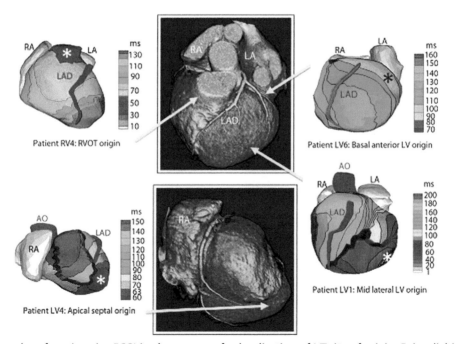

Fig. 9. Examples of noninvasive ECGI isochrone maps for localization of VT site of origin. Epicardial isochrone maps are shown for 4 patients, with earliest epicardial activation marked with an asterisk. Sites of origin determined by electrophysiologic study are indicated under the ECGI maps. Yellow arrows point to VT origin on a representative CT scan. AO, aorta; LA, left atrium; LAD, left anterior descending coronary artery; LV, left ventricle; RA, right atrium; RVOT, right ventricular outflow tract. (*From* Wang Y, Cuculich PS, Zhang J, et al. Noninvasive electroanatomic mapping of human ventricular arrhythmias with electrocardiographic imaging (ECGI). Sci Transl Med 2011;3:4; with permission.)

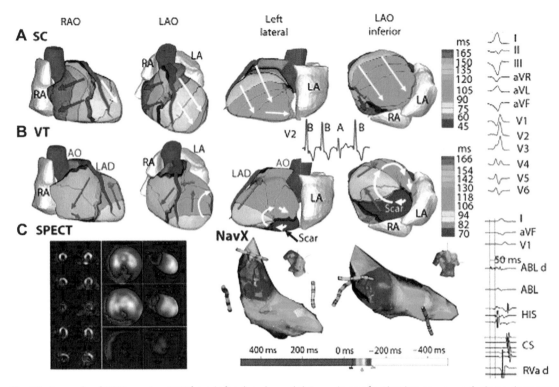

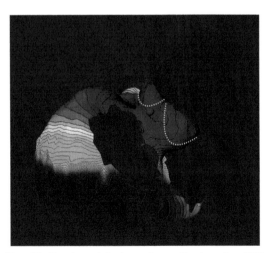

Fig. 10. Example of ECGI reentrant VT from inferobasal scar. (*A*) Four views of activation sequence during a sinus capture (SC) beat (*blue* on the V2 ECG). Arrows indicate direction of the activation wave fronts. (*B*) Activation sequence during VT beats (*red* on the V2 ECG). White arrows indicate a clockwise lateral loop (left lateral and left anterior oblique inferior views); purple arrows show propagation into the RV in a counterclockwise fashion. (*C*) (*Left*) Single-photon emission CT (SPECT) images showing a scar at the inferobasal LV region (*blue*). (*Right*) Limited invasive endocardial map of VT activation (*red*, early; *blue*, late). (*Right column*) (*Top*) Twelve-lead surface ECG during VT. (*Lower*) Ablation catheter signals. The earliest electrogram signal is seen at the inferoseptal border zone, 50 milliseconds before the onset of the surface QRS. ABL d, bipolar electrogram at the distal ablation catheter; CS, coronary sinus; HIS, AV junction/His bundle; LAO, left anterior oblique view; RAO, right anterior oblique view; RVa d, right ventricular apex. (*From* Wang Y, Cuculich PS, Zhang J, et al. Noninvasive electroanatomic mapping of human ventricular arrhythmias with electrocardiographic imaging (ECGI). Sci Transl Med 2011;3:6; with permission.)

The accuracy of ECGI mapping has been demonstrated over a wide range of origins, and distinguishes focal from macro-reentrant mechanisms with a high degree of spatial resolution in the range of 6 mm.[7] Because of the linkage to the CT scan specific to the patient under study, the maps correlate with the anatomy of the individual patient. There are limitations with this approach, which records epicardial activation, because there are differences in activation between the endocardium and epicardium. This activation is affected by thickness of the myocardium, fiber orientation, and scar. Nonetheless, it provides useful supplemental information to facilitate endocardial mapping.

Fig. 11. Focal ventricular ectopy. Noninvasive ECG mapping demonstrating early activation from the region of the aortic cusps. (*Courtesy of* Meleze Hocini, MD, Bordeaux, France.)

FOCAL AND MACRO-REENTRANT ATRIAL ARRHYTHMIAS

The evolution of ablation procedures has encompassed a variety of sustained atrial arrhythmias

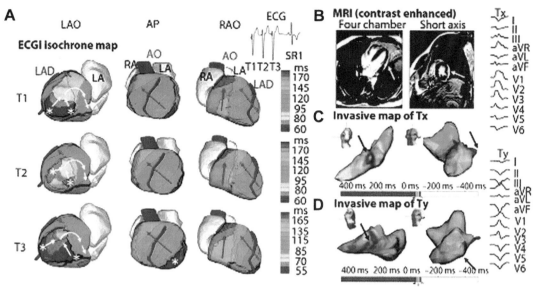

Fig. 12. Example of ECGI of reentrant VT in LV lateral wall infiltrative cardiomyopathy. (*A*) ECGI isochrone map. Activation patterns for 3 consecutive VT beats (T1, T2, and T3). ECGI identified 2 distinct areas of early epicardial activation (*white asterisks*), which differed from beat to beat. The propagation pattern varied somewhat depending on the relative contribution of the 2 sources, but for all beats, the wave front turned clockwise and propagated to the LV lateral base with a high degree of curvature (*white arrows*), where it reached a line of block in the infero-lateral base. Rose arrows show direction of wave front propagation in other regions of the epicardium. (*B*) Gadolinium-enhanced MRI revealed a patch of myocardial enhancement in the lateral LV (*white arrows*), consistent with focal myocarditis or cardiac sarcoid. (*C*) Invasive electroanatomic map created during the presenting VT (arbitrarily named Tx). The region of earliest activation is shown by black arrows. (*D*) Invasive electroanatomic map created during a different VT (arbitrarily named Ty) after initial ablation at the site of earliest activation. The earliest activation (*black arrows*) is shifted more apically. (*Right*) Twelve-lead ECGs of 2 VT morphologies (Tx and Ty). AP, anterior-posterior view; SR1, first sinus rhythm beat after VT. (*From* Wang Y, Cuculich PS, Zhang J, et al. Noninvasive electroanatomic mapping of human ventricular arrhythmias with electrocardiographic imaging (ECGI). Sci Transl Med 2011;3:7; with permission).

that depend on either focal or reentrant mechanisms. Ablation of premature atrial complexes is uncommon because they tend not to be associated with severe symptoms; however, in some patients triggers of atrial fibrillation that arise outside of the pulmonary veins may be important, but are difficult to map and often cannot be induced reliably enough to map accurately. Early attempts to map atrial arrhythmias using ECGI were directed toward the focal mechanism because the specific anatomic location could be confirmed by endocardial mapping and compared with results of ECGI; they were later followed by studies of reentry.[9,34]

Fig. 13 shows 3-dimensional ECGI images that were recorded in a patient with a history of rheumatic heart disease and mitral valve commissurotomy who had undergone a prior pulmonary vein antral isolation and subsequently developed a focal atrial tachycardia.[9] An epicardial breakthrough (local potential minimum) was recorded high in the left atrium near the septum. Results

of ECGI mapping showed a good correlation with endocardial electroanatomic mapping and the site of ablation. Another example, shown in **Fig. 14**, illustrates a focal atrial tachycardia with centrifugal activation from the base of the left atrial appendage.[34] This image was recorded with the same prototype system that was used in **Fig. 11**.

Additional studies using the ECM system (CardioInsight) evaluated the efficacy in both focal mechanisms of atrial tachycardia and macro-reentry involving cavotricuspid isthmus-dependent, perimitral, and left atrial roof–dependent reentry.[34] **Fig. 15** shows cavo-tricuspid isthmus-dependent counterclockwise rotation around the tricuspid valve. **Fig. 16** is an example of perimitral atrial flutter, and **Fig. 17** shows macro-reentrant roof-dependent left atrial flutter. ECM correctly diagnosed the mechanism of atrial tachycardias in 92% of patients with focal or macro-reentrant mechanisms that were located in either the right or left atrium. The main limitation was that the system did not provide direct

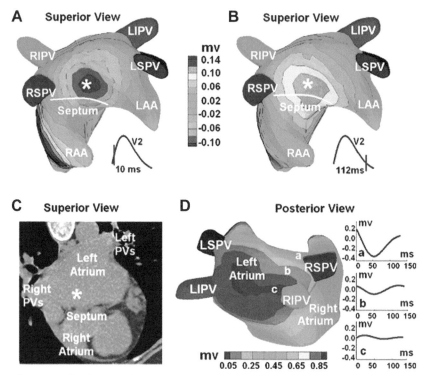

Fig. 13. ECGI 3-dimensional voltage and electrogram maps of focal atrial tachycardia (AT). (*A, B*) Atrial epicardial potential maps at 10 and 112 milliseconds after the onset of the surface P wave. Panel *A* captures the epicardial breakthrough pattern during activation, and *B* shows the repolarization pattern with reverse polarity. The white asterisk indicates the site of earliest activation as predicted by ECGI. (*C*) ECGI-determined earliest activation site (*white asterisk*) on a CT image of the atria. (*D*) Electrogram magnitude map (peak-to-peak) reconstructed by ECGI (*posterior view*). The dark blue area represents a region of low-magnitude electrograms, indicating a scar region. Three electrograms selected from a nonscar region (*a*) and from the scar region (*b, c*) are shown. Location of the low-magnitude electrograms is consistent with prior pulmonary vein (PV) isolations and left atrial substrate modification. LAA, left atrial appendage; LIPV, left inferior PV; LSPV, superior PV; RAA, right atrial appendage; RIPV, right inferior PV; RSPV, right superior PV. (*From* Wang Y, Cuculich PS, Woodard PK, et al. Focal atrial tachycardia after pulmonary vein isolation: noninvasive mapping with electrocardiographic imaging (ECGI). Heart Rhythm 2007;4:1082; with permission.)

mapping of the septum; however, a septal source often can be deduced by analyzing the location and timing of epicardial activation near the interatrial groove.

ATRIAL FIBRILLATION

The physiology of human atrial fibrillation has been difficult to study because of the need for simultaneous recordings in both atria and sophisticated computer algorithms to reconstruct complex electrical activation. Moreover, the physiology of atrial fibrillation may differ depending on whether it is recorded in an animal model or human. In patients the atria may be affected by hypertension, myopathies, valvular heart disease, or other comorbidities. There is compelling

clinical and experimental evidence that long duration of atrial fibrillation is associated with more complex physiology. It also seems to be dependent on both anatomic barriers and progressive changes at a cellular level that affect cell-to-cell conduction and refractoriness. The multiple wavelet hypothesis proposed by the seminal work of Moe and Abildskov[35] has been widely accepted for many years, yet it was based on a canine model of atrial fibrillation dependent on vagal nerve stimulation, which provided the basis for computer modeling. Allessie and colleagues[36] promoted the leading circle concept for atrial fibrillation that was independent of anatomic barriers or areas of conduction block, and found evidence of 4 to 6 simultaneous randomly circulating wavelets in

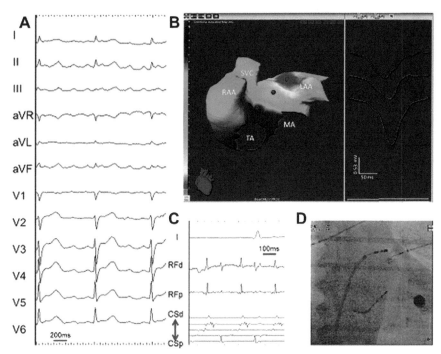

Fig. 14. Focal left AT. (*A*) A 12-lead ECG of clinical tachycardia. (*B*) An ishochronal activation electrocardiomap of a basal left atrial appendage source centrifugal AT. The morphology of the virtual unipolar electrogram at the source displays typical QS morphology. (*C*) Intracardiac electrograms from the lateral left atrium and coronary sinus recorded during ablation of the left atrial source centrifugal AT. (*D*) Posteroanterior fluoroscopic image showing the location of intracardiac catheters. LAA, left atrial appendage; MA, mitral annulus; RAA, right atrial appendage; SVC, superior vena cava; TA, tricuspid annulus. (*From* Shah AJ, Hocini M, Xhaet O, et al. Validation of novel 3-dimensional eletrocardiographic mapping of atrial tachycardias. Invasive mapping and ablation. A multicenter study. J Am Coll Cardiol 2013;62:895; with permission.)

Langendorff-perfused atria with an acetylcholine infusion. Other studies based on different animal models have raised the possibility that diverse mechanisms are involved.[37–41] Lee and colleagues[41] performed high-density mapping during vagal nerve stimulation in the canine heart, and concluded that multiple foci of varying cycle lengths and duration induced wave fronts that merged or collided without random wave fronts of reentry.

Early epicardial mapping of induced atrial fibrillation obtained from humans in the operating room used 156 electrodes applied to the right atrial free wall, the posterior left atrial tissue beneath the posterior septum and pulmonary veins, and the transverse sinus to map the anterior right and left atrial tissue.[42,43] These studies commonly observed multiple dynamic wave fronts interacting with changing arcs of conduction block and slow conduction. Sometimes transient macro-reentry was observed without anatomic obstacles, but these circuits were transient and unstable with

cycle lengths of 200 to 240 milliseconds. Although most circuits were centered in the left atrium, others were recorded in the right atrium. More recent intraoperative mapping studies of patients with chronic atrial fibrillation that used 404 epicardial electrodes demonstrated 2 patterns.[44] In one, parts of the atria demonstrated short regular cycle lengths that could be consistent with a driver with irregular activation of the rest of the atria. The second pattern showed no regions of regular activation.

Current strategies for ablation of atrial fibrillation have focused on elimination of the triggers of atrial fibrillation or modification of the substrate required to prevent atrial fibrillation, yet complex activation sequences that occur during atrial fibrillation cannot be interpreted by single-point endocardial mapping.

Preliminary studies showing the complexity of mapping electrical activation during atrial fibrillation highlighted individual variation and differences between patients with paroxysmal and persistent

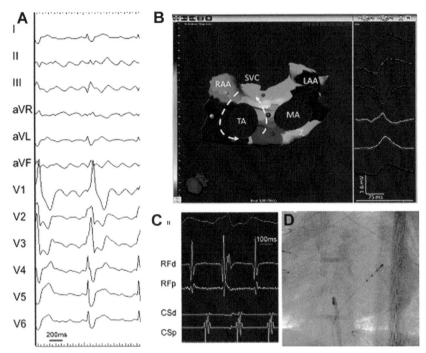

Fig. 15. Cavotricuspid isthmus-dependent AT. (*A*) A 12-lead ECG of clinical tachycardia from a patient who previously underwent extensive ablation for atrial fibrillation (AF). (*B*) An isochronal activation electrocardiomap of counterclockwise cavotricuspid isthmus-dependent AT. Typically, the interatrial groove is activated from below upward followed by sequential activation of the right atrial free wall from above downward. The left atrial breakthroughs at the coronary sinus and the Bachmann bundle result in septal to lateral activation of the anterior and posterior left atrium. The morphology of the virtual unipolar electrograms displayed from atrial sites distributed around the tricuspid annulus concurs with this activation pattern. The color of the unipolar electrogram corresponds to the color of the spot marked on the biatrial geometry. On the color scale, the earliest activation site is red and the latest is purple. The color map shows 160 milliseconds of activation. The cycle length here is 244 milliseconds. The remainder of the cycle length is within the slow conduction zone (cavotricuspid isthmus), on either side of which purple meets red. (*C*) Intracardiac electrograms from the isthmus and coronary sinus recorded during the ablation of cavotricuspid isthmus-dependent AT. (*D*) Posteroanterior fluoroscopic image showing the location of intracardiac catheters. LA, left atrial appendage; MA, mitral annulus; RAA, right atrial appendage; SVC, superior vena cava; TA, tricuspid annulus. (*From* Shah AJ, Hocini M, Xhaet O, et al. Validation of novel 3-dimensional eletrocardiographic mapping of atrial tachycardias. Invasive mapping and ablation. A multicenter study. J Am Coll Cardiol 2013;62:892; with permission.)

atrial fibrillation.[7] In aggregate, multiple wavelets are observed in a high percentage of patients (92%), and focal mechanisms can be demonstrated in pulmonary and nonpulmonary vein origins. **Fig. 18** shows a posterior view of the left atrium recorded during atrial fibrillation, and demonstrates a reentrant wave front recorded at 2 points in time that enters the posterior left atrium through a protected isthmus. **Fig. 19** shows the spectrum of complexity of AF (the reader is referred to Cuculich and colleagues[7] for actual ECGI maps and movies of complex activation in persistent atrial fibrillation). There are statistical differences in the number of wavelets and focal mechanisms when paroxysmal, persistent, and

long-standing persistent atrial fibrillation are compared. The observation that paroxysmal atrial fibrillation has less complex wavelets and fewer focal mechanisms helps to explain why the success rate of catheter ablation is higher in patients with paroxysmal atrial fibrillation as opposed to atrial fibrillation of long-standing duration. Although these patterns are often repetitive in patients with paroxysmal atrial fibrillation, the repetition of patterns decreases with the complexity of atrial fibrillation.

These observations are concordant with panoramic mapping of atrial fibrillation reported by Haissaguerre and colleagues,[45] who recorded reconstructed unipolar electrograms during atrial

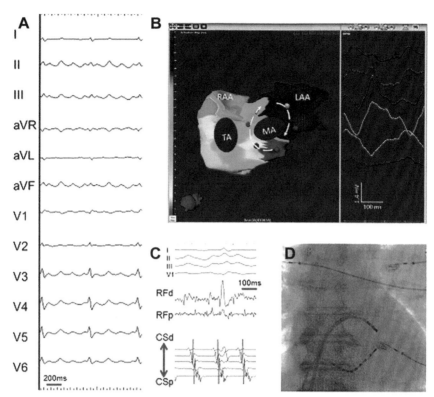

Fig. 16. Perimitral AT. (*A*) A 12-lead ECG of clinical tachycardia. (*B*) An isochronal activation electrocardiomap of clockwise perimitral AT. Typically, the coronary sinus and contiguous posteroinferior left atrium are activated from a lateral to septal direction, and the Bachmann bundle activation proceeds in the opposite direction, covering almost the entire tachycardia cycle length. The morphology of the virtual unipolar electrograms displayed from 6 atrial sites distributed around the mitral annulus confirms the activation pattern. The right atrial free wall is typically activated from above downward during perimitral AT. The cavotricuspid isthmus is activated laterally (toward the right atrial free wall) from the septum (coronary sinus ostium level) without substantial conduction delay confirming the bystander role of the right atrium in perimitral AT. (*C*) Intracardiac electrograms from the lateral mitral isthmus and coronary sinus recorded during the ablation of perimitral AT. (*D*) Posteroanterior fluoroscopic image showing the location of intracardiac catheters. LAA, left atrial appendage; MA, mitral annulus; RAA, right atrial appendage; TA, tricuspid annulus. (*From* Shah AJ, Hocini M, Xhaet O, et al. Validation of novel 3-dimensional eletrocardiographic mapping of atrial tachycardias. Invasive mapping and ablation. A multicenter study. J Am Coll Cardiol 2013;62:893; with permission.)

fibrillation using an array of 252 body surface electrodes (CardioInsight) registered to a noncontrast CT scan. As shown in **Fig. 20**, this study observed continuously changing reentrant patterns lasting a median 2.6 rotations. Although the wave fronts varied over time and space, repetitive wave-front patterns and focal drivers were observed and provided a potential target for ablation. Approximately 70% of the reentrant patterns and focal drivers were recorded in the left atrium. As with the prior study reported by Cuculich and colleagues,[7] the number of targeted drivers increased from a median of 2 to 6 in relation to the duration of atrial fibrillation. Ablation in these regions terminated

75% of persistent and 15% of long-standing atrial fibrillation, but the probability of termination decreased sharply in patients with atrial fibrillation of longer than 6 months' duration.

Limitations of the mapping system developed by CardioInsight are that electrograms recorded from tissue that is heavily scarred with low-amplitude signals requires careful interpretation. The mapping system reconstructs electrograms relative to the epicardial surface, so activation of the septum can be inferred but wave fronts in the depth of the septum are not recorded directly.

Overall, animal and human studies testify to the complexity of atrial fibrillation that depends on

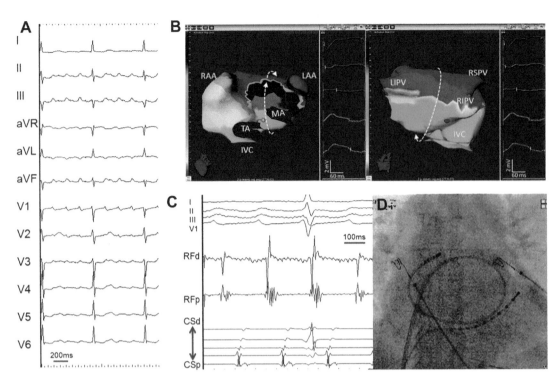

Fig. 17. Left atrial roof-dependent AT. (*A*) A 12-lead ECG of clinical tachycardia. (*B*) Ishochronal activation of an electrocardiomap of a typical macro-reentrant roof-dependent AT. The below to upward activation of the anterior wall of the left atrium is shown on the left and the top to bottom activation of the posterior left atrium is shown on the right. The bystander right atrial free wall is activated from above downward. The entire tachycardia cycle length is covered along the AT circuit, and the morphologies of the virtual unipolar electrograms displayed from 5 atrial sites distributed along the trajectory of the macro-reentry concur with this activation pattern. (*C*) Intracardiac electrograms from the left atrial roof and coronary sinus recorded during the ablation of roof-dependent AT. (*D*) Posteroanterior fluoroscopic image showing the location of the intracardiac catheters. IVC, inferior vena cava; LAA, left atrial appendage; MA, mitral annulus; RAA, right atrial appendage; TA, tricuspid annulus. (*From* Shah AJ, Hocini M, Xhaet O, et al. Validation of novel 3-dimensional eletrocardiographic mapping of atrial tachycardias. Invasive mapping and ablation. A multicenter study. J Am Coll Cardiol 2013;62:894; with permission.)

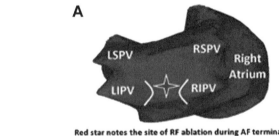

Red star notes the site of RF ablation during AF termination.
White lines note the proposed isthmus.

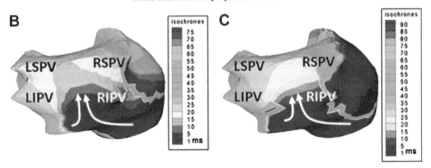

Fig. 18. Noninvasive ECGI of AF using a critical isthmus in the posterior left atrium during AF radiofrequency ablation. (*A*) Posterior view of the atria with a red star marking the location of the ablation that terminated AF. (*B*, *C*) ECGI ishochrone maps during AF at 2 separate time points immediately before successful ablation. For both images a wave front enters the posterior left atrium (*white arrows*) through a protected isthmus. LIPV, left inferior PV; LSPV, left superior PV; PV, pulmonary vein; RIPV, right inferior PV; RSPV right superior PV. (*From* Cuculich PS, Wang Y, Lindsay BD, et al. Noninvasive characterization of epicardial activation in humans with diverse atrial fibrillation patterns. Circulation 2010;122:1367; with permission.)

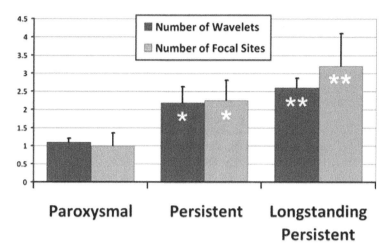

Fig. 19. Increasing complexity of AF stratified by clinical classification of paroxysmal, persistent, and long-standing persistent AF. With increasing AF duration, ECGI imaged more focal sites and wavelets (analysis of variance: for wavelet $P = .11$; focal sites $P = .031$). Asterisk denotes $P<.05$ compared with paroxysmal. Double asterisk denotes $P<.05$ compared with both paroxysmal and persistent. (*Adapted from* Cuculich PS, Wang Y, Lindsay BD, et al. Noninvasive characterization of epicardial activation in humans with diverse atrial fibrillation patterns. Circulation 2010;122:1370; with permission.)

chronicity, the extent of fibrosis, and other factors. The development of improved ablation strategies and other therapeutic approaches will depend on improved understanding of the physiology of atrial fibrillation gained by these sophisticated mapping systems.

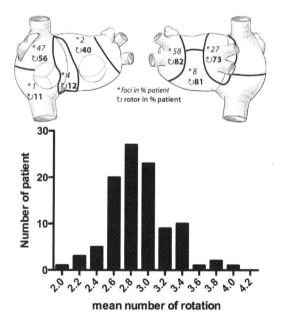

Fig. 20. Persistent AF. (*Top*) Distribution of drivers (focal breakthroughs, *asterisk*; reentry events, *curved arrows*) in 7 regions is reported as the percentage of patients. For example, 82% of the 103 patients had repetitive reentries, and 58% had repetitive focal breakthroughs in the left PV–appendage region. (*Bottom*) Distribution of the mean number of rotations in 103 patients. (*From* Haissaguerre M, Hocini M, Denis A, et al. Driver domains in persistent atrial fibrillation. Circulation 2014;130:533; with permission.)

REFERENCES

1. Plonsey R, Barr RC. Bioelectricity—a quantitative approach. 3rd edition. New York: Springer; 2007.
2. Barr RC, Ramsey M III, Spach MS. Relating epicardial to body surface potential distributions by means of transfer coefficients based on geometry measurements. IEEE Trans Biomed Eng 1977;24:1–11.
3. Ramanathan C, Ghanem RN, Jia P, et al. Noninvasive electrocardiographic imaging for cardiac electrophysiology and arrhythmia. Nat Med 2004;10:422–8.
4. Jia P, Ramanathan C, Ghanem RN, et al. Electrocardiographic imaging of cardiac resynchronization therapy in heart failure: observations of variable electrophysiologic responses. Heart Rhythm 2006; 3:296–310.
5. Silva JN, Ghosh S, Bowman TM, et al. Cardiac resynchronization therapy in pediatric congenital heart disease: insights from noninvasive electrocardiographic imaging. Heart Rhythm 2009;6:1178–85.
6. Ghosh S, Silva JN, Canham RM, et al. Electrophysiologic substrate and intraventricular left ventricular dyssynchrony in nonischemic heart failure patients undergoing cardiac resynchronization therapy. Heart Rhythm 2011;8:692–9.
7. Cuculich PS, Wang Y, Lindsay BD, et al. Noninvasive characterization of epicardial activation in humans with diverse atrial fibrillation patterns. Circulation 2010;122:1364–72.
8. Wang Y, Schuessler RB, Damiano RJ, et al. Noninvasive electrocardiographic imaging (ECGI) of scar-related atypical atrial flutter. Heart Rhythm 2007;4:1565–7.
9. Wang Y, Cuculich PS, Woodard PK, et al. Focal atrial tachycardia after pulmonary vein isolation: noninvasive mapping with electrocardiographic imaging (ECGI). Heart Rhythm 2007;4:1081–4.
10. Wang Y, Cuculich PS, Zhang J, et al. Noninvasive electroanatomic mapping of human ventricular

arrhythmias with electrocardiographic imaging. Sci Transl Med 2011;3:98ra84.

11. Colli Franzone P, Guerri L, Taccardi B, et al. The direct and inverse potential problems in electrocardiology: numerical aspects of some regularization methods and application to data collected in isolated dog heart experiments. Lab Anal Numerica CNR report. 1979; 222.

12. Rudy Y, Messinger-Rapport BJ. The inverse problem in electrocardiography: solutions in terms of epicardial potentials. Crit Rev Biomed Eng 1988;16:215–68.

13. Tikhonov AN, Arsenin VY. Solution of ill-posed problems. New York: John Wiley and Sons; 1977.

14. Ramanathan C, Jia P, Ghanem RN, et al. Noninvasive electrocardiographic imaging (ECGI): application of the generalized minimal residual (GMRes) method. Ann Biomed Eng 2003;31:981–94.

15. Oster HS, Taccardi B, Lux RL, et al. Noninvasive electrocardiographic imaging: reconstruction of epicardial potentials, electrograms and isochrones, and localization of single and multiple electrocardiac events. Circulation 1997;96:1012–24.

16. Oster HS, Taccardi B, Lux RL, et al. Electrocardiographic imaging: noninvasive characterization of intramural myocardial activation from inverse reconstructed epicardial potentials and electrograms. Circulation 1998;97:1496–507.

17. Burnes JE, Taccardi B, Rudy Y. A noninvasive imaging modality for cardiac arrhythmias. Circulation 2000;102:2152–8.

18. Burnes JE, Taccardi B, MacLeod RS, et al. Noninvasive electrocardiographic imaging of electrophysiologically abnormal substrate in infarcted hearts: a model study. Circulation 2000;101:533–40.

19. Ghanem RN, Burnes JE, Waldo AL, et al. Imaging dispersion of myocardial repolarization ii. noninvasive reconstruction of epicardial measures. Circulation 2001;104:1306–12.

20. Ghanem RN, Jia P, Ramanathan C, et al. Noninvasive electrocardiographic imaging (ECGI): comparison to intraoperative mapping in patients. Heart Rhythm 2005;2:339–54.

21. Abraham WT, Fisher WG, Smith AL, et al. Cardiac resynchronization in chronic heart failure. N Engl J Med 2002;346:1845–53.

22. Fung JW, Yu CM, Yip G, et al. Variable left ventricular activation pattern in patients with heart failure and left bundle branch block. Heart 2004;90:17–9.

23. Durrer D, Van Dam RT, Freud G, et al. Total excitation of the isolated human heart. Circulation 1970;41:899–912.

24. Ramanathan C, Jia P, Ghanem R, et al. Activation and repolarization of the normal human heart under complete physiological conditions. Proc Natl Acad Sci U S A 2006;103:6309–14.

25. Auricchio A, Fantoni C, Regoli F, et al. Characterization of left ventricular activation in patients with heart failure and left bundle-branch block. Circulation 2004;109:1133–9.

26. Bradley DJ, Bradley EA, Baughman KL, et al. Cardiac resynchronization and death from progressive heart failure: a meta-analysis of randomized controlled trials. JAMA 2003;289:730–40.

27. Cuculich PS, Zhang J, Wang Y, et al. The electrophysiologic cardiac ventricular substrate in patients after myocardial infarction: noninvasive characterization with electrocardiographic imaging. J Am Coll Cardiol 2011;58:1893–902.

28. Rudy Y. Noninvasive electrocardiographic imaging of arrhythmogenic substrates in humans. Circ Res 2013;112:863–74.

29. Thibault B, Ducharme A, Harel F, et al. Left ventricular versus simultaneous biventricular pacing in patients with heart failure and a QRS complex ≥120 milliseconds. Circulation 2011;124:2874–81.

30. Ghosh S, Rhee EK, Avari JN, et al. Cardiac memory in WPW patients: noninvasive imaging of activation and repolarization before and after catheter ablation. Circulation 2008;118:907–15.

31. Hocini M, Shah AJ, Cochet H, et al. Noninvasive electrocardiomapping facilitates previously failed ablation of right appendage diverticulum associated life-threating accessory pathway. J Cardiovasc Electrophysiol 2013;24:583–5.

32. Wang Y, Li L, Cuculich PS, et al. Electrocardiographic imaging of ventricular bigeminy in a human subject. Circ Arrhythm Electrophysiol 2008;1:74–5.

33. Zhang J, Desouza KA, Cuculich PS, et al. Continuous ECGI mapping of spontaneous VT initiation, continuation, and termination with antitachycardia pacing. Heart Rhythm 2013;10:1244–5.

34. Shah AJ, Hocini M, Xhaet O, et al. Validation of novel 3-dimensional eletrocardiographic mapping of atrial tachycardias. Invasive mapping and ablation. A multicenter study. J Am Coll Cardiol 2013;62:889–97.

35. Moe GK, Abildskov JA. Atrial fibrillation as a self-sustaining arrhythmia independent of focal discharge. Am Heart J 1959;58:59–70.

36. Allessie MA, Lammers WJ, Bonke FI, et al. Experimental evaluation of Moe's multiple wavelet hypothesis of atrial fibrillation. In: Zipes DP, Jalife J, editors. Cardiac electrophysiology and arrhythmias. New York: Grune & Stratton; 1985. p. 265–75.

37. Scheussler RB, Grayson TM, Bromberg BI, et al. Cholinergically mediated tachyarrhythmias induced by a single extrastimulus in the isolated canine right atrium. Circ Res 1992;71:1254–67.

38. Kumagai K, Khrestian C, Waldo AL. Simultaneous multisite mapping studies during induced atrial fibrillation in the sterile pericarditis model: Insights into the mechanism of its maintenance. Circulation 1997;95:511–21.

39. Skanes AC, Mandapati R, Berenfeld O, et al. Spatiotemporal periodicity during atrial fibrillation

in the isolated sheep heart. Circulation 1998;98: 1236–48.

40. Mandapati R, Skanes A, Chen J, et al. Stable micro-reentrant sources as a mechanism of atrial fibrillation in the isolated sheep heart. Circulation 2000;101: 194–9.

41. Lee S, Sahadevan J, Khrestian C, et al. High density mapping of atrial fibrillation during vagal nerve stimulation in the canine heart: restudying the Moe hypothesis. J Cardiovasc Electrophysiol 2013;24:328–35.

42. Cox JL, Canavan TE, Schuessler RB, et al. The surgical treatment of atrial fibrillation. II. Intraoperative electrophysiologic mapping and description of the electrophysiologic basis of atrial flutter and atrial fibrillation. J Thorac Cardiovasc Surg 1991;101: 406–26.

43. Ferguson TB Jr, Schuessler RB, Hand DE, et al. Lessons learned from computerized mapping of the atrium. Surgery for atrial fibrillation and flutter. J Electrocardiol 1993;26(Suppl):210–9.

44. Sahadevan J, Kyungmoo R, Peltz L, et al. Epicardial mapping of chronic atrial fibrillation in patients. Preliminary observations. Circulation 2004;110:3293–9.

45. Haissaguerre M, Hocini M, Denis A, et al. Driver domains in persistent atrial fibrillation. Circulation 2014; 130:530–8.

Computation and Projection of Spiral Wave Trajectories During Atrial Fibrillation: A Computational Study

CrossMark

Ali Pashaei, PhD[a,b,*], Jason Bayer, PhD[a,b],
Valentin Meillet, MSc[a,b], Rémi Dubois, PhD[a,b],
Edward Vigmond, PhD[a,c]

KEYWORDS

- Cardiac electrophysiology • Atrial fibrillation • Body surface potential map • Phase mapping

KEY POINTS

- No strong relation was found between dominant frequency and phase singularity location for meandering rotors.
- Phases computed with the Hilbert transform method can produce spurious phase information if cells return to rest for extended periods between beats.
- Complexity of activity is increased on the convex hull of the atria.
- Loss of frequency content on the surface may limit the reconstruction of epicardial activity.

Videos of spiral wave trajectories during atrial fibrillation accompany this article at http://www. cardiacep.theclinics.com/

INTRODUCTION

Phase analysis[1] has become a useful tool for the interpretation of fibrillatory activity.[2] It provides an amplitude-independent manner in which to characterize and visualize dynamic data, especially important for inverse mapping. This tool is helpful during fibrillation when activity is complicated because of wavefront interactions, leading to constant fractionation and collision. Beyond using phase statistics to simply classify arrhythmia,

phase singularities (PSs) represent organizing centers and, thus, have become targets for ablation therapy.[3,4]

The concept that underlies phase is that the instant within the cell cycle can be characterized by an angle, which can be considered as time relative to the action potential onset normalized to the duration of the cellular action potential. It is convenient to take phase 0 as rest, just before the cell begins to depolarize, and the complete return to

This work was supported through the Investment of the Future grant, ANR-10-IAHU-04, from the government of France through the Agence National de la Recherche. A. Pashaei is supported by the Agence National de Recherche grant no ANR-13-MONU-0004-02. J. Bayer is supported by the Whitaker International Program administered by the Institute for International Education.

[a] LIRYC Electrophysiology and Heart Modelling Institute, University of Bordeaux, PTIB–Campus Xavier, Arnozan, Avenue du Haut Lévêque, Bordeaux 33600, France; [b] Inserm U1045, Cardiothoracic Research Center, 146 rue Léo-Saignat, Bordeaux Cedex 33076, France; [c] Bordeaux Institute of Mathematics UMR 5251, University of Bordeaux, 351 cours de la Libération, Talence 33405, France
* Corresponding author. IHU LIRYC, PTIB–Campus Xavier Arnozan, Avenue du Haut Lévêque, Pessac 33600, France.
E-mail address: ali.pashaei@ihu-liryc.fr

cardiacEP.theclinics.com

rest as occurring at a phase angle of 2π. Several methods have been proposed to calculate phase, including time embedding[1] and the Hilbert transform.[5] Furthermore, the center of a functional reentry is identified by its core, which is a point of PS, meaning the phase at the point is itself undefined, but all phases are found encircling the point. These PSs may be located by spatial analysis of phase maps but may also be determined directly by the intersection of isolines.[6] However, which of the methods performs best for atrial fibrillation (AF) has yet to be resolved.

The relationship between activity on the atrial epicardium and activity recorded on the torso body remains to be fully elucidated. A recent study[7] has found, using simplified geometries for the atria and torso, that the number of PSs detected on the body surface potential map is reduced compared with the number found on the atrial surface. This finding could present a theoretic limitation of inverse mapping,[8] because filtering by the body could limit accurate reconstruction of potentials on the epicardium, and, hence, PSs. The study also found that when filtered at the correct frequency, the location of the dominant frequency (DF) on the torso is related to the position of the DF on the atria.

This is a computational study with 2 aims. The first is to compare the number and position of PSs as determined by 3 methods: time embedding, filament detection, and the Hilbert transform. The second aim is to see if a relationship exists between DF and PSs on different surfaces, starting from the epicardium and expanding to the torso, to understand how phase information is affected by volume conduction in a geometrically realistic situation.

METHODS
Spiral Waves in Two Dimensions

To study phase computation in a simpler geometry, spiral waves were induced in a 2-cm × 2-cm sheet discretized at 100 μm into a triangular finite element mesh. Simulations were performed with the CARP software[9] using a monodomain formulation with zero flux boundary condition using the Courtemanche human atrial cell model.[10] Cell properties inside a circular domain of radius 5 mm in the center of slab were changed to double intrinsic action potential duration (APD) (by increasing the background calcium current 5-fold and halving the rapid potassium current) to attract the phase singularity. Tissue conductivity was isotropic and set to 0.236 s/m everywhere (conduction velocity about 0.2 m/s). Reentry was initiated with a typical cross-field S1S2 protocol, as

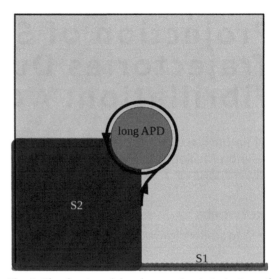

Fig. 1. The sheet model and approximate trajectory of the rotor core around the region with long APD (*dark gray*). The S1 stimulus along the bottom edge was applied at time 0 and S2 at 250 milliseconds.

shown in **Fig. 1**. Simulations were run for 400 milliseconds to generate 1 spiral wave following a trajectory on the edge of circular domain starting at time 250 milliseconds. Results were output every 1 millisecond. **Fig. 1** shows the schematic and approximate spiral wave core trajectory.

Computer Model of Atria and Atrial Fibrillation

A computed tomography (CT)-derived bilayer computer model of the atria was used, which incorporated structural and conductive elements, including left and right atria, discrete connection paths between the right and left atria, fiber orientation, pectinate muscles, and inflow vessels. A modified Courtemanche human atrial ionic model was used.[11] Tissue conductivities were set to closely match clinically measured values. Full details of the model are available in Ref.[12] Reentry was induced by an ectopic focus centered around the pulmonary vein delivered at 270 milliseconds after a normal beat originating from the sinoatrial node. The reentry, which developed, was sustained and persisted for the length of the simulation, 3.4 seconds. Output was sampled every 5 milliseconds.

To observe changes with distance from the epicardium, 10 surfaces were interpolated from the atria to the torso, on which phase maps were computed from surface potentials (**Fig. 2**). To begin, the convex hull of the atria (ie, the minimal elastic surface enclosing the atria) was generated using MeshLab (http://meshlab.sourceforge.net/).

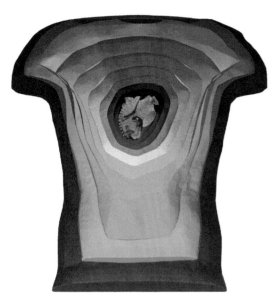

Fig. 2. Ten surface meshes, ranging from the convex hull of the atria to the torso surface. A coronal plane in the middle of the torso shows the placement of the atria. Each layer is indicated by a different color.

A torso mesh of a male was obtained from CT and discretized into a set of 17,592 triangles (mean edge size 9.7 mm). The torso was homogeneous and isotropic, with no organs. To interpolate the surfaces between the convex hull and the torso, a freely available tool called volMorph was used.[13]

Transmembrane voltages computed during reentry were used to compute extracellular potentials. Each surface was considered separately, with potentials on a surface calculated by solving the following equation:

$$(H_B + I/2)\, \varphi_b = \varphi_a$$

where φ_b is the vector of unknown boundary surface potentials, H_B is the dipole matrix computing the potentials produced on the boundary by the boundary sources, φ_a is the potential produced by the heart sources on the body surface, and I is the identify matrix. This solution implies no flux conditions. Furthermore, the solution was constrained so that the average potential on the exterior boundary surface was zero. The boundary element method was used with first order triangles, and the resulting system of equations solved by single value decomposition with the Elemental Distributed Matrix library.[14] The number of unknowns ranged from 1256 on the convex hull to 8798 on the torso. Phase maps were constructed from the surface potentials by low pass filtering at 15 Hz, zero averaging each signal, and then applying the Hilbert transform (**Fig. 3**).

IDENTIFICATION OF SPIRAL WAVES

In this article, only activity in thin layers is considered, and, thus, spiral waves in the form of rotors that rotate about PSs (ie, rotor cores) are discussed. Two main approaches for locating PSs were studied.

Filament Detection

All phases are present in the neighborhood surrounding a PS. Thus, to identify this point, we used a modified method of Fenton and Karma[6] by determining the intersection of transmembrane voltage isolines. **Fig. 3**A provides a two-dimensional (2D) demonstration of the intersection points of isolines of membrane voltage at −10, −20, −30, −40, and −50 mV (black lines) with the isoline of voltage extremum $dV_m/dt = 0$ (white line). Isolines were computed by interpolation of the nodal values on the edges. This method could be performed only on the atrial surface.

Phase Analysis

PSs can also be determined by examining maps of phase. The transmembrane voltage signal was converted to phase by 1 of the 2 methods outlined later, for each instant in time. Each point in the mesh cycles between 0 and 2π. PSs are then identified as the points around which all phases are present at 1 point in time, which is equivalent to the line integral of the phase around the PS being nonzero (see **Fig. 3**D). The contours of integration were taken as the edges defining the elements that constituted the computational domain.

Time embedding

A phase space representation of the signal can be produced by plotting the signal versus a time-delayed version of itself. If the delay is properly chosen, the phase space point follows a simple loop, as in **Fig. 3**B. The phase is computed as the rotation of the phase space point around a center point. To fit this center, we used a Voronoi point (ie, the center of the maximum inscribed circle inside the loop), as shown in **Fig. 3**C. Again, the transmembrane voltage is required for this technique.

Discrete-time Hilbert transform

Discrete-time Hilbert transform is the most general method for phase determination, because any time series can be used. A discrete-time Hilbert transform was applied,[5] which generates a complex signal from which a phase can be calculated. To avoid error associated with signal notch, a band-pass Butterworth filter with upper frequency cutoff, f_c, is used to remove high-frequency

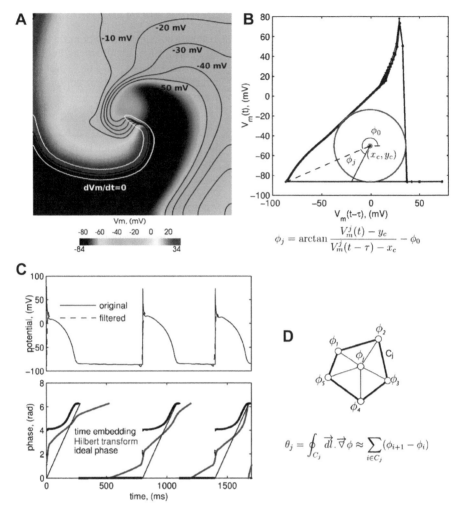

Fig. 3. Phase singularity detection. (*A*) Filament detection computes the intersection between $dV_m/dt = 0$ (*white line*) and isocontour of a selected potential value (*black lines*). Isopotentials from −50 to −10 mV are shown. Colors represent transmembrane voltage. (*B*) Phase state trajectory for time-embedding method. The red circle is the largest inscribed circle for determining the center, whereas the blue line shows the angle offset for the zero phase point. (*C*) Phase-based methods are applied in 2 steps. (*Upper panel*) The original time series was low pass filtered. (*Bottom panel*) Phase computed using Hilbert transform (*red*) or time embedding with a lag of 3 milliseconds (*blue*) compared with the ideal signal (*black*). (*D*) Spatial domain to compute the line integral of phase change around points in the domain. Triangles represent elements of the computational mesh.

components of the potential signal. The upper panel in **Fig. 3**B shows the original and filtered signal. The red line in the plot of the lower panel shows the phase change computed from Hilbert transform technique for the signal. Here, the black line shows the expected phase value, which varies linearly each cycle over time regardless of the cycle length.

Definition of Trajectories

A trajectory of a rotor was defined as the continuous movement of a PS. If the PS is allowed to move at a maximum speed of C, then between

frames, a PS can move at most a distance of $C\Delta t$ along a trajectory, where Δt is the output period. Thus, PSs were analyzed in adjacent output frames, and if the 2 PSs were separated by less than this distance, they were assumed part of the same trajectory. The number of both PSs and trajectories over the course of the simulation were counted.

RESULTS
Sheet Simulations

To gauge the different phase calculation methods, the Hilbert transform method was first compared with time embedding for the simple case of a sheet paced periodically along 1 edge (see **Fig. 3**C). In both cases, the phase was a monotonic function, but neither showed the linear increase, as was expected. When there was a significant pause between pacing beats, the Hilbert transform method extended the phase over a longer period than that of the action potential, rather than following the period of pacing. For rapid pacing (ie, a stimulus period less than that of the APD at rest), the method performed as expected. The time-embedding method followed the action potential and showed a zero phase after the return of the action potential to rest.

Under reentry conditions shown in **Fig. 1**, a single rotor rotation was observed, as shown with potential map in Video 1 (available online at http://www.cardiacep.theclinics.com/). **Fig. 4** shows trajectories computed from filament detection, Hilbert transform, and time-embedding phase analysis methods, respectively. Video 2 (available online at http://www.cardiacep.theclinics.com/) shows the trajectory for these cases mapped on the rotor dynamics in 3 methods, respectively. To study the sensitivity of the methods to processing parameters, 6 different values were used for each method, covering a reasonable spectrum of values. For the filament detection method, the isoline of the membrane voltage, Vm, was changed from -10 to -60 mV. In a similar fashion, for the Hilbert transform method, the upper

frequency cutoff parameter, f_c, was changed with values of 10 to infinity. For the time-embedding method, trajectories were computed for time lags of 2 to 25 milliseconds. The PS statistics are shown in **Table 1**. All methods showed a similar question mark–shaped trajectory, as expected, corresponding to a PS being formed at the intersection of the recovery and S2 fronts, and then moving to follow the boundary of the long APD region. The phase methods were more similar to each other, with an additional initial descending segment that was more separated from the subsequent ascending portion. Also, the phase methods had additional PSs, especially along the edges, but these were not consistent between the 2 phase methods. Additional postprocessing was applied to remove PSs along the edges, and these were not considered.

The choice of isoline did not much affect filament detection. For higher voltages, there were a couple of brief initial PSs, which were not present at lower voltages. Looking at **Table 1**, voltages between -30 and -60 mV performed similarly. For the Hilbert transform, a certain degree of filtering was necessary, but severe filtering less than 20 Hz performed badly. All cutoff frequencies between 20 and 120 gave similar results. Time embedding performed very poorly for very small or very large lags, with lags between 3 and 7 milliseconds working best.

Phase analysis methods generated more PSs and disconnected trajectories and provided more

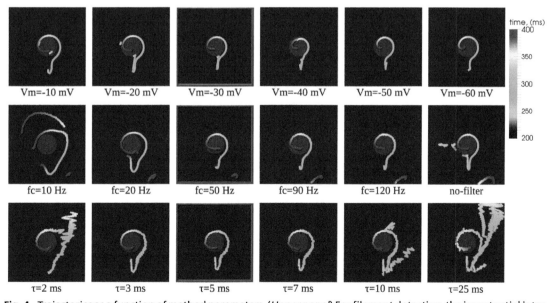

Fig. 4. Trajectories as a function of method parameters. (*Upper panel*) For filament detection, the isopotential intersection. (*Middle panel*) For the Hilbert transform, low pass cutoff frequencies. (*Lower panel*) For time embedding, time lags were varied. Cases indicated by the red border were used for further comparison. Video 2 (available online at http://www.cardiacep.theclinics.com/) shows the trajectory for these cases mapped on the rotor dynamics in 3 methods, respectively. Color indicates the time that the PS was detected.

Table 1
Number of detected PSs and number of trajectories for the 3 methods as a function of method parameters

Parameter (Unit)	Filament Detection						Hilbert Transform						Time Embedding				
	Isopotential, Vm (mV)						Cutoff Frequency, fc (Hz)						Time Lag, τ (ms)				
Value	−10	−20	−30	−40	−50	−60	20	50	70	90	120	No filter	2	3	5	7	10	25
Number of PSs	176	168	155	152	150	150	208	213	216	217	215	258	199	151	151	151	249	460
Number of trajectories	3	2	1	1	1	1	2	2	2	2	2	4	2	1	1	1	4	7

consistent shapes (ie, those that were closer to the circle defining the boundary between short and long APD).

To compare the spatial position of the PSs detected, the distance between the PSs computed by the different methods was plotted (cases with red border in **Fig. 4**) along the primary trajectory, shown in **Fig. 5**. The true PS positions are not known, so only relative positions can be compared. The closest correspondence was between filament detection and the Hilbert transform, which was in the order of 300 mm after the reentry moved to the edge of the circle. The furthest separation was between filament and time embedding, which was about 1 mm. The difference between the time embedding and Hilbert was in between.

Spiral Waves on Atria

During simulation of AF in the atria, the trajectory of the spiral cores was mapped on the surface mesh of the epicardium. **Fig. 6** and Video 3 (available online at http://www.cardiacep.theclinics.com/) show the trajectory for the anterior and posterior views of the PS trajectories over 3000 milliseconds. In addition, the DF of each point was computed and is shown in **Fig. 6** along with the trajectories. Rotors were not fixed but meandered over the surface of the left atrium, spending time near the pulmonary veins (see Video 3). The DFs ranged from 4 to 6 Hz, with the highest-frequency region being near the left superior pulmonary vein. Although the rotors passed through that region, it was not a site of persistent anchoring. The left inferior pulmonary vein was the site of frequent rotor meandering but still showed a low DF. A spatial relationship between DF and rotor trajectory was not apparent.

Spiral Waves on Different Layers

The Hilbert transform phase analysis method, with a cutoff of 15 Hz, was applied to the surface potentials to compute PSs on each of 10 layers. **Fig. 7A** and Video 4 (available online at http://www.cardiacep.theclinics.com/) show the trajectory of the spiral cores on different layers with solid lines. The number of PSs and trajectories are given for each layer in **Fig. 8**. The largest number of PSs was detected on the convex hull, which is closest to the heart, even more than was detected on the heart itself. Otherwise, the number of PSs and trajectories decreased with distance from the epicardium. The number of PSs was approximately 50 times greater than the number of rotors, and this was constant across all surfaces. The trajectories on the surface covered very large regions and were not localized. Video 5 (available online at http://www.cardiacep.theclinics.com/) shows how the PS points on the torso are related to the electrogram map. Comparing the power spectra of the convex hull (see **Fig. 7B**) and the torso (see **Fig. 7C**), it is seen that the high frequencies are filtered out of the torso potentials. There are 3 main closely spaced peaks in the first, fundamental lobe, which are present in all layers, and the harmonics dropped out by the fourth surface. Correspondingly, the dominant frequencies are lower on the torso, with the highest-frequency region under the right armpit. On the convex hull, the highest-frequency regions were located on the right atrium, which did not correspond to the dominant frequencies on the epicardium.

Discussion

This study is the first to simulate AF in realistically shaped atria and calculate the phase on a geometrically correct torso. Several ways to calculate

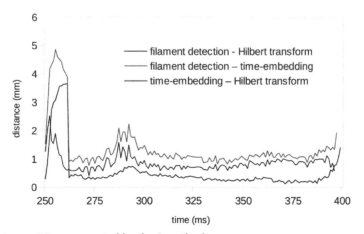

Fig. 5. Distances between PSs as computed by the 3 methods.

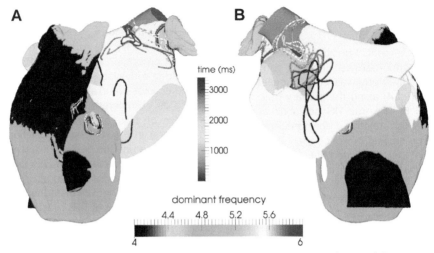

Fig. 6. Trajectory of the rotor cores projected on to DF map of the atrial epicardium in (*A*) anterior and (*B*) posterior views. PS trajectories are drawn as lines with a blue-white-red color scale, signifying the time at which the PS was located at a point. Dominant frequencies are indicated by the rainbow color scale. Note that the inferior vena cava was not active, because they contain no myocytes.

phase were also compared, and the correlation between phase trajectories and dominant frequencies was examined. The analysis performed highlights several considerations when applying dominant frequencies and phase singularity location in a clinical context, to determine ablation sites.

HILBERT TRANSFORM

The Hilbert transform applies a sinusoidal decomposition based on the fundamental frequency, which tends to be that of stimulation and not that of the action potential. During reentry, when cells are continually activated, with no pause in

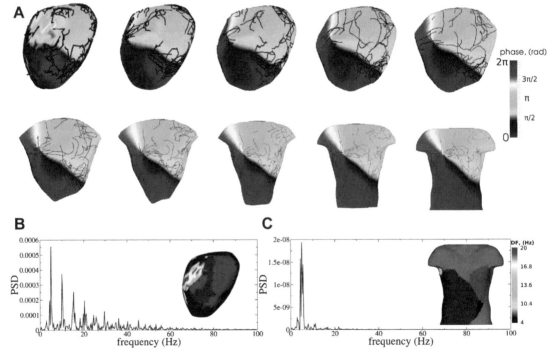

Fig. 7. (*A*) Phase distribution on the 10 surfaces at time 3400 milliseconds. Lines indicate phase trajectories. (*B*) Typical power spectral densities at a point on the convex hull with the DF map inset. (*C*) Typical torso power spectral density with inset torso DF map. Dominant frequencies for (*B*) and (*C*) are indicated by the color bar on the right.

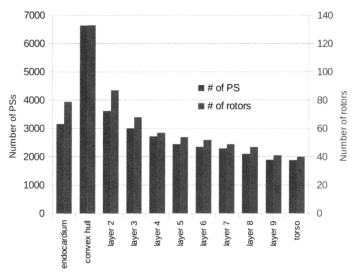

Fig. 8. Number of detected singularity points and trajectories for different layers.

between, the Hilbert transform computes a phase as expected. However, if there is a significant pause, the Hilbert transform interpolates the phase between the excitation times, which means that the phase during rest is nonzero. This situation may lead to an inaccurate or spurious identification of a PS, and hence, a point clinically ineffective for ablation. This shortcoming also applies to more elaborate phase reconstruction algorithms using the Hilbert transform, like that of Kuklik and colleagues.[15] Assuming that the system is continually excited, the Hilbert transform can be used when there are only excitation data, as is the case with surface electrograms recorded during fibrillation.

FILAMENT-BASED VERSUS PHASE-BASED METHODS

Using both filament detection and phase analysis methods on action potential waveforms, the trajectory tracking algorithm captured the expected trajectory in the 2D sheet. There were some dissimilarities in the predicted trajectories from the different methods. The filament detection method predicts a smoother and continuous trajectory. On the other hand, the phase analysis method provides consistent trajectories for different input parameters, but some unwanted trajectories appeared, in particular near the edges.

More PSs are detected with phase analysis methods, with the Hilbert transform detecting the highest. Many of them were aligned on the boundaries. Some of these observations can be explained by reexamining the basis for detection of PS in these methods: in phase analysis, methods look for points surrounded by all phases, whereas filament detection is based on intersection of

isolines. Any change in this isoline (Vm), relocates the crossing point with the isoline of voltage extremum, hence changing PS location and trajectory. On the other hand, there is not direct correlation between the upper-band cutoff frequency and location of the PS in phase analysis methods. The filament detection algorithm has the advantage that it is simple to implement and is computationally less expensive. It predicts the trajectory, with fewer artifacts. However, at some points, it detects more than 1 root at the intersection of isolines. This factor can be fulfilled using a distance thresholding between detected PS that merges those closer than a certain distance in each time frame. Also, because of derivative operator in filament detection, more sensitivity can be expected to noise.

The difference in trajectory between any of the methods was less than a millimeter, and thus, smaller than the area affected under an ablation catheter.

OPTIMAL PARAMETER VALUES

With the filament detection method, changing the isovoltage value altered the shape of the trajectory. Isoline of −30 mV was used as the optimum parameter in the slab model.

The Hilbert transform method was improved when a Butterworth filter was used. In practice, cutoff frequencies of about 15 Hz were used for tracking the singularity points on tissue layers. Lower cutoff frequencies show a more linear phase map in normal transmembrane voltage signals, but at the cost of increased artifacts. Studying residuals of action potentials for different cutoff frequency confirms that the used frequency is in range of optimum values.

The time-embedding method provides relatively consistent trajectories for different values of lag, except in low values, in which trajectory is noisy. A lag of about 5 milliseconds was found to be optimal, which is close to that used previously.[1] The method is known to fail if no loop in phase space is present or the center point falls outside the phase loop. However, this method works best with signals that change over their entire cycle, a criterion not fulfilled by electrograms.

CONVEX HULLS

The convex hull showed more PSs than on the epicardium, as well as retaining the high-frequency content. The increased number of PSs is because of the condition that topological charge over the entire surface must be equal to zero. Besides a PS producing net topological charge, the integral of the topological charge around the boundary of a zone of inexcitability may also be nonzero, as in the case of anatomic reentry around a valve opening or vein. Thus, a PS on the convex hull may not be a PS on the atria but may be the topological charge around an opening.

Additional complexity seen on the convex hull may also result from field interaction, in which the enclosing hull overlies distinct concave surfaces, as near the atrial junction and around the pulmonary veins. The atrial model has 2 layers, and the activities may be discordant.

These considerations highlight that caution must be used when looking at reconstructed PSs on the atria. The surfaces used for reconstruction can contain features of convex hulls and are not completely separate atria with holes and discrete connections, so spurious PSs may be generated.

COMPARISON WITH PREVIOUS WORK

Rodrigo and colleagues[7] recently performed a study of the relationship between the location of PSs and the location of the DF. Several observations from our study need discussion in this context. As their study showed, the number of PSs decreases with distance from the epicardium. However, several important distinctions need to be made.

First, we simulated reentry on actual atrial and torso geometry, which is more complicated than spheres, given the discrete coupling implemented between the left and right atria, as well as the many perforations. A sphere resembles more the convex hull of our study (see earlier discussion). It is to be expected that the sphere has more PSs than the atria. In light of the conservation of topological charge, we are reticent to classify a PS on the torso (a closed surface) as true or mirror,[7] because PSs must be created in pairs and the force compelling creation of one equally compels creation of the second.

Rotors in our simulations were not stationary, as indicated by the trajectories. The dominant frequencies were not strongly associated with regions where the PSs spent most of the time. Furthermore, regions in the atria showed discrete changes in frequency as opposed to a smooth transition. It is not clear which frequency to take as the one for filtering. Under the conditions of this study, it is difficult to argue that localization of dominant frequencies by PS identification is meaningful or clinically useful. Ablation based on DF has generally not proved effective.[16–18] However, not all AF is the same, and a strong correlation between DF and PS location for stationary rotors may exist.[19]

LIMITATIONS

We have chosen a particular set of parameters to attain AF. Modifying parameters to create a stationary rotor could change the results. Algorithms can be highly sensitive to noise and the parameters used, such as type of filtering, cutoff frequency, and sampling rate. Phase mapping is robust, in that we have found that PSs are always present, albeit in different locations, regardless of the processing to create the phase map. Fourier transform analysis, whether for the computation of Hilbert transforms or dominant frequencies, assumes stationarity, which does not hold in general during AF.

SUMMARY

The Hilbert transform performs well if the heart is continuously excited. No relationship was found between phase singularity location and DF. Frequency content was filtered as the signal moved away from the heart surface, suggesting a limit for the reconstruction of epicardial potentials from torso measurements.

VIDEOS

Videos related to this article can be found online at http://dx.doi.org/10.1016/j.ccep.2014.11.001.

REFERENCES

1. Gray RA, Pertsov AM, Jalife J. Spatial and temporal organization during cardiac fibrillation. Nature 1998; 392(6671):75–8. http://dx.doi.org/10.1038/32164.
2. Umapathy K, Nair K, Masse S, et al. Phase mapping of cardiac fibrillation. Circ Arrhythm Electrophysiol 2010; 3(1):105–14. http://dx.doi.org/10.1161/CIRCEP.110.853804.

3. Haissaguerre M, Hocini M, Shah AJ, et al. Noninvasive panoramic mapping of human atrial fibrillation mechanisms: a feasibility report. J Cardiovasc Electrophysiol 2013;24(6):711–7. http://dx.doi.org/10.1111/jce.12075.

4. Narayan SM, Shivkumar K, Krummen DE, et al. Panoramic electrophysiological mapping but not electrogram morphology identifies stable sources for human atrial fibrillation: stable atrial fibrillation rotors and focal sources relate poorly to fractionated electrograms. Circ Arrhythm Electrophysiol 2013; 6(1):58–67. http://dx.doi.org/10.1161/CIRCEP.111.977264.

5. Bray MA, Wikswo JP. Considerations in phase plane analysis for nonstationary reentrant cardiac behavior. Phys Rev E Stat Nonlin Soft Matter Phys 2002;65(5 Pt 1):051902.

6. Fenton F, Karma A. Vortex dynamics in three-dimensional continuous myocardium with fiber rotation: filament instability and fibrillation. Chaos 1998; 8(1):20–47.

7. Rodrigo M, Guillem MS, Climent AM, et al. Body surface localization of left and right atrial high-frequency rotors in atrial fibrillation patients: a clinical-computational study. Heart Rhythm 2014; 11(9):1584–91. http://dx.doi.org/10.1016/j.hrthm.2014.05.013.

8. Rudy Y. Noninvasive imaging of cardiac electrophysiology and arrhythmia. Ann N Y Acad Sci 2010;1188:214–21. http://dx.doi.org/10.1111/j.1749-6632.2009.05103.x.

9. Vigmond EJ, Hughes M, Plank G, et al. Computational tools for modeling electrical activity in cardiac tissue. J Electrocardiol 2003;36(Suppl):69–74. Available at: http://www.ncbi.nlm.nih.gov/pubmed/14716595.

10. Courtemanche M, Ramirez RJ, Nattel S. Ionic mechanisms underlying human atrial action potential properties: insights from a mathematical model. Am J Physiol 1998;275(1 Pt 2):H301–21.

11. Krummen DE, Bayer JD, Ho J, et al. Mechanisms of human atrial fibrillation initiation: clinical and computational studies of repolarization restitution and activation latency. Circ Arrhythm Electrophysiol 2012;5(6):1149–59. http://dx.doi.org/10.1161/CIRCEP.111.969022.

12. Labarthe S, Bayer J, Yves Coudiere Y, et al. A bilayer model of human atria: mathematical background, construction, and assessment. Europace 2014;16: iv21–9.

13. Treece G, Prager R, Gee A. Volume-based three-dimensional metamorphosis using sphere-guided region correspondence. Vis Comput 2001;17(7): 397–414. http://dx.doi.org/10.1007/s003710100113.

14. Poulson J, Marker B, van de Geijn RA, et al. Elemental: a new framework for distributed memory dense matrix computations. ACM Trans Math Softw 2013;39(2):1–24. http://dx.doi.org/10.1145/2427023.2427030.

15. Kuklik P, Zeemering S, Maesen B, et al. Reconstruction of instantaneous phase of unipolar atrial contact electrogram using a concept of sinusoidal recomposition and Hilbert transform. IEEE Trans Biomed Eng 2014. http://dx.doi.org/10.1109/TBME.2014.2350029.

16. Elvan A, Linnenbank AC, van Bemmel MW, et al. Dominant frequency of atrial fibrillation correlates poorly with atrial fibrillation cycle length. Circ Arrhythm Electrophysiol 2009;2(6):634–44.

17. Jarman JW, Wong T, Kojodjojo P, et al. Spatiotemporal behavior of high dominant frequency during paroxysmal and persistent atrial fibrillation in the human left atrium. Circ Arrhythm Electrophysiol 2012; 5(4):650–8. http://dx.doi.org/10.1161/CIRCEP.111.967992.

18. Katritsis DG, Pantos I, Efstathopoulos EP. Catheter ablation of atrial fibrillation guided by electrogram fractionation and dominant frequency analysis. Expert Rev Cardiovasc Ther 2011;9(5):631–6.

19. Guillem MS, Climent AM, Millet J, et al. Noninvasive localization of maximal frequency sites of atrial fibrillation by body surface potential mapping. Circ Arrhythm Electrophysiol 2013;6(2):294–301. http://dx.doi.org/10.1161/CIRCEP.112.000167.

Analysis of Cardiac Fibrillation Using Phase Mapping

Richard H. Clayton, PhD[a],*, Martyn P. Nash, PhD[b]

KEYWORDS

- Cardiac arrhythmia • Ventricular fibrillation • Atrial fibrillation • Mapping • Reentry • Phase analysis

KEY POINTS

- Phase mapping provides a way to represent the electrical activation–recovery cycle of cardiac tissue and can be used for the robust identification of reentry.
- The calculation of phase angle involves several processing steps, which must be implemented carefully to obtain a good estimate of phase.
- Preprocessing of electrograms, especially those recorded from the atrium, is important to obtain a robust estimate of phase angle.

INTRODUCTION

Although the detailed mechanisms that sustain fibrillation in the human heart continue to be debated,[1–3] it is well accepted that the irregular waveform seen on a surface electrocardiogram during atrial (AF) and ventricular (VF) fibrillation arises from an irregular and constantly changing activation sequence. Electrical activity in the myocardium during fibrillation can be mapped with electrode arrays in the in situ heart[4–6] using voltage-sensitive fluorescent dyes in the isolated heart.[7–9] Recent studies indicate the potential utility of body surface electrodes for mapping atrial activity.[10,11] All of these modalities show complex and often irregular activity. Interpreting these signals is difficult, and this is an obstacle both to understanding the basic science underlying these clinically important arrhythmias and to developing strategies for clinical interventions, such as atrial ablation.

The idea of using phase to represent electrical activation and recovery in the heart was developed in the 1980s, with a focus on identifying the timing of abnormal beats capable of initiating reentry.[12] These ideas were then extended to identify functional reentry during fibrillation from singularities in phase maps[13] obtained from optical mapping with voltage-sensitive fluorescent dyes. This approach had the important advantage that it was not necessary to construct maps of activation times, as in earlier studies of arrhythmia mechanisms,[14] which can be difficult in areas of block and slow conduction.

The focus of this review is to explain the benefits and limitations of phase mapping for both basic science and clinical applications by describing the concepts of phase analysis and methods for obtaining phase from voltage measurements, as well as the potential hazards associated with different approaches. There is a focus on applications in the human heart, and the aim is to complement other recent reviews that concentrate on interpolation and phase mapping,[15] and phase analysis in simulations.[16]

The authors have no conflicts of interest.
[a] Insigneo Institute for *in-silico* medicine and Department of Computer Science, University of Sheffield, Regent Court, 211 Portobello Street, Sheffield S1 4DP, UK; [b] Auckland Bioengineering Institute and Engineering Science, University of Auckland, Uniservices House, Level 7, Room 439-715, 70 Symonds Street, Auckland 1010, New Zealand
* Corresponding author.
E-mail address: r.h.clayton@sheffield.ac.uk

cardiacEP.theclinics.com

MECHANISMS OF REENTRY AND FIBRILLATION IN THE HEART

Reentry describes a circulating wave of electrical activation that continually propagates into recovering tissue, resulting in rapid and self-sustaining electrical activity.[3] Reentry is an important mechanism in both AF and VF.

During reentry, activation rotates around a core, which may be an anatomic obstacle or a region of functional block. The center of rotation is surrounded by tissue in all parts of the activation–recovery cycle. In the thick-walled ventricles, the center of rotation is a filament around which the activation wavefront is wrapped as a scroll wave. If the filament is aligned across the ventricular wall, then it is observed as a center of rotation, or rotor, on the ventricular epicardium. However, other filament configurations are possible, and these include ring-shaped filaments that give rise to spreading circular activation waves on the epicardial surface.[16] The more complex anatomy of the thin-walled atria offers more opportunities for anatomic reentry. Atrial filaments are comparatively short, and so the centers of rotation effectively behave as points rather than filaments.

In early studies that provided direct evidence of reentry, activation times derived from unipolar electrograms obtained with contact electrodes were used to determine the progression of an activation wave around a reentrant circuit.[17–19] Subsequent studies of tortuous activation sequences during VF also used this approach,[20] but beyond illustrative examples it was difficult to quantitatively describe the reentrant mechanism.

The advent of cardiac mapping based on signals from voltage-sensitive fluorescent dyes offered a way to image electrical activation of the myocardial surface with much greater spatial resolution,[21,22] and this has now become a standard technique in the experimental setting. Phase analysis was developed to interpret the high spatial resolution information that can be gained from these measurements,[13] and offers an alternative way to detect and quantify reentry than approaches based on activation times. The fluorescent dyes used in optical mapping experiments are toxic, and so cannot be used in the in situ human heart. As a result, the approaches developed for transforming optical action potentials into phase have been adapted for use with electrograms.[5,15]

BASIC PRINCIPLES OF PHASE ANALYSIS

The idea of using phase to represent a repetitive or oscillatory process is commonly used in the study of other physical systems, where the state of the system is represented as a phase angle. In the example shown in **Fig. 1**, the behavior of a simple

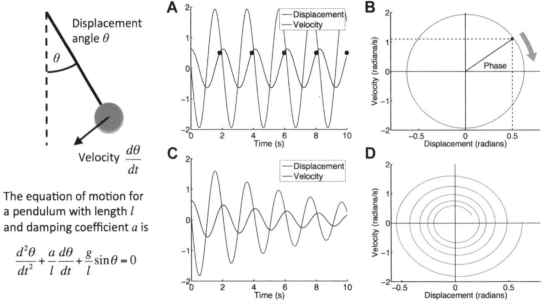

Fig. 1. Motion of a simple pendulum with and without damping described using the equation shown. (A) Time series plot of displacement (*blue*) in radians, and velocity (*red*) in radians s^{-1} for an undamped pendulum of length 1 m, with initial displacement of $\pi/5$ radians. (B) State-space plot of velocity plotted against displacement, where red and blue lines show zero velocity and zero displacement, respectively. Red and blue dashed lines indicate point in the pendulum oscillations where displacement is 0.5 radians. These points are shown for each cycle in A. (C, D) corresponding plots for a damped pendulum.

pendulum is simulated, and the state of the pendulum is described by its displacement (angle from the vertical) and velocity (rate of change of displacement). The displacement and velocity of an undamped pendulum can be shown in time series plots (see **Fig. 1**A), or by plotting velocity against displacement (see **Fig. 1**B). This second plot is a state-space plot, where at each instant the relative values of the 2 state variables, the velocity and the displacement of the pendulum, characterize the state of the system. In these state-space plots, we use W to denote the variable on the vertical axis and V to denote the variable on the horizontal axis.

For the oscillating pendulum, the displacement is greatest when the velocity is zero, and vice versa. Thus in the time series plots of **Fig. 1**A, peaks in displacement (V) precede peaks in velocity (W) by one-quarter of the period; therefore, the state-space trajectory is circular and clockwise, with 1 orbit corresponding with 1 period of the pendulum.

The relative values of V and W at any instant can be expressed as phase, which is the angle subtended by the point in state-space and one of the axes. In this example, the phase was calculated from the arc-tangent of velocity over displacement, and for the point shown in **Fig. 1**B this angle is the arc-tangent of 1.092/0.5, which is 1.14 radians. This phase angle seems to be smaller on the figure because the range of values shown on the vertical axis is nearly 4 times as great as the range on the horizontal axis. Typically, phase calculations use the *atan2* function, which is available in most programming environments. For a clockwise rotation, *atan2* yields a phase angle ranging from 0 radians at 3 o'clock to $-\pi$ radians at 9 o'clock, and then from π radians at 9 o'clock back to 0 radians at 3 o'clock. Phase therefore varies in the range $-\pi$ radians to π radians ($-180°$ to $180°$). If phase is plotted as a time series, there are discontinuities as the trajectory passes through 9 o'clock, causing the phase angle to jump from π radians to $-\pi$ or vice versa.

With no damping, the pendulum continues to oscillate for an infinite time; each period traces a single orbit of the phase trajectory, and phase varies over the range of $[-\pi, \pi]$ radians. If damping is included in the pendulum simulation, the amplitude of oscillations gradually decreases (see **Fig. 1**C), and the trajectory becomes a spiral (see **Fig. 1**D). Despite the decrease in amplitude, and providing that the displacement is not zero, it remains possible to represent the oscillations as phase. If, instead of a simulation, measurements of velocity and displacement were made, then the phase could still be obtained, even if these

measurements included some noise. Thus, representing cardiac activation and recovery as phase can avoid the problem of assigning activation times to noisy and low-amplitude electrograms. However, this representation requires careful choices of the state variables, as well as the origin in state-space, for the phase representation to be reliably meaningful.

TRANSFORMATION INTO PHASE PLANE

The prerequisites for phase analysis are therefore 2 state variables, W and V, that yield a trajectory that orbits a single point when plotted against each other. Ideally, peaks in one of these state variables should precede peaks or troughs in the other by around one-quarter of a cycle, so that the state-space trajectory is circular.

For phase mapping in cardiac electrophysiology, the state variable, V, is usually a signal related to electrical activity, such as an optical action potential or electrogram. In simulations, the second state variable, W, can be chosen to be a model variable that represents recovery.[23,24] However, for experimental data where only optical action potentials or electrograms can be measured, a careful choice is needed, because an unsuitable choice can lead to errors in the phase calculation, and ambiguities in interpretation of the results.

Models of cardiac cell and tissue electrophysiology are useful tools to explore these considerations, because they provide a ground truth against which different approaches can be evaluated. The simulations used in the subsequent section are described in detail in a previous publication.[25] Briefly, a single reentrant wave was initiated in a 2-dimensional sheet of simulated human ventricular tissue, with cellular electrophysiology described by a model of human ventricular electrophysiology,[26] adapted such that a single reentrant wave broke up into multiple wavelets, as is typically observed during fibrillation.[5]

A time series of action potentials recorded from 1 location in the sheet is shown in **Fig. 2**A. Early studies of phase mapping in cardiac electrophysiology used an optical action potential $v(t)$ as V, and a time delayed representation $v(t-\tau)$ as W,[13,23] where τ is a constant time delay. This approach is known as time delay embedding, and **Fig. 2**B shows a trajectory in state-space obtained with this approach, using the time series in **Fig. 2**A delayed by $\tau = 20$ ms. The red circle in **Fig. 2**B indicates an origin (V^*, W^*), with coordinates given by the mean of each of the state variables, which can be used to calculate the phase angle $atan2([W - W^*]/[V - V^*])$. These choices of delay and origin yield an anticlockwise trajectory.

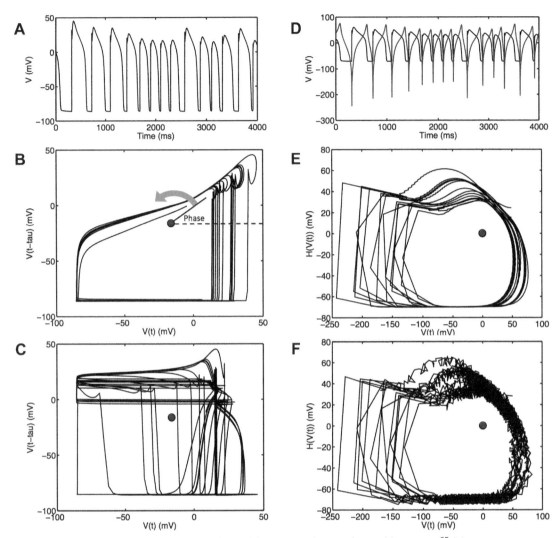

Fig. 2. (*A*) Time series of action potentials derived from a simulation of unstable reentry.[25] (*B*) State-space representation of time series in *A* with time delay embedding and a time delay of 20 ms. The red circle denotes an origin at the mean value of voltage, and the green arrow indicates that the direction of trajectory in state-space is anticlockwise. (*C*) Representation of time series in *A* with time delay embedding, and a time delay of 150 ms. (*D*) Time series of action potentials as in *A* (*blue*), combined with the Hilbert transform of this time series (*red*). (*E*) State-space representation of time series in *D*, where the state variable on the vertical axis is the Hilbert transform. Red circle denotes origin at (0,0). (*F*) Representation as shown in *E*, but with the addition of noise.

However, the trajectory passes close to the origin point, and this can lead to difficulties with the phase angle calculation. For example, if the voltage time series was distorted by experimental noise, then there is the possibility that the trajectory would pass below the origin point during some cycles. The consequence would be that the phase angle would not vary correctly through the range [−π, π] radians for each cycle. The choice of this origin is therefore important for correct identification of phase, but it may need to be determined empirically if time delay embedding

is used. In this example, moving the origin so that *W** is fixed at −50 mV moves it closer to the center of the trajectory.

The other important choice in this approach is the time delay parameter τ, and a good choice is critical for correct identification of phase. **Fig. 2C** illustrates the effect of changing τ from 20 to 150 ms. In the latter case, not all of the activation–recovery cycles in the time series lead to a complete rotation about the origin. The way that this affects the phase calculation is considered in the next section.

For experimental data, a suitable time delay is the time at which the signal and its delayed version are most independent, and this can be calculated as the first minimum of the autocorrelation function, which is typically around one-quarter of the fibrillation cycle length.[13,23] In simulations, a much shorter time delay, equivalent to the duration of the action potential upstroke, provides a good choice.[23,27] As with the origin, an empirical choice of delay that gives the best trajectory may be necessary.

Time delay embedding can be effective, especially in simulations,[28] providing that both the time delay and the origin point are chosen carefully. An advantage is that only 2 snapshots of electrical activity are required to calculate phase at a particular point in time. An alternative embedding technique is to use an integral of electrogram voltage over a sliding window as the second state variable W.[29] In the more general literature, the derivative of V has been described,[30] but for cardiac electrophysiology numerical estimates of the derivative can be very sensitive to noise.

The most widely used alternative to time delay embedding is the Hilbert transform,[31] which automatically generates a second state-space variable W that is time shifted relative to V by one-quarter of a cycle at each time point. This is equivalent to time delay embedding with a variable time delay that is optimized for each point of the time series. The red trace in **Fig. 2**D shows the Hilbert transform of the data shown in **Fig. 2**A, and **Fig. 2**E shows the state-space representation, where the Hilbert transform is plotted against the time series data. The trajectory is more circular than the trajectory obtained with time delay embedding (see **Fig. 2**B), and is much more robust when the time series is corrupted by adding some artificial noise (see **Fig. 2**F). If the mean of the time series signal is set to zero by subtracting the mean from every point before applying the Hilbert transform, then the mean of the Hilbert transform is also zero, and so the origin in state-space can be set at (0,0).

The Hilbert transform is therefore a robust approach. However, a time series for each point in space (electrode or pixel from optical mapping) is needed. Small amplitude signals or those with sharp deflections can still result in unreliable phase calculations; hence, amplitudes of the time series signals may need to be increased where necessary.[31]

IDENTIFICATION OF PHASE SINGULARITIES

The tip of a reentrant wave is surrounded by tissue in all parts of the activation–recovery cycle, and at this point it is not possible to specify the phase.

Thus the center of rotation in reentry is described as a phase singularity (PS), and lies at the point at which lines of equal phase converge. **Fig. 3** illustrates clockwise reentry and the identification of a PS in the model described earlier. The snapshot in **Fig. 3**A shows simulated membrane voltage in a large (25 × 25 cm), 2-dimensional sheet of tissue, 1000 ms after initiation of reentry. **Fig. 3**B shows the phase map of this snapshot, where the phase of each point in the simulation was calculated using time delay embedding with a delay of 20 ms as illustrated in **Fig. 2**B. The lines of equal color converge on a single PS, which is located close to the center of the figure, and is highlighted by a white circle and by the arrow in the inset, which shows an expanded view of the pixels at the PS core.

The precise location of a PS can be identified because the pixels that surround it show a complete phase change of 2π. In this example, the 4 pixels surrounding the PS in the inset have phase angles of approximately $-\pi$ radians (blue), $+1.5$ radians (orange), $+1$ radians (yellow), and -1 radians (turquoise). This property can be used to automate the identification of PS in a phase map either by examining the change in phase around each pixel[23] or by using a convolution kernel.[27] In **Fig. 3**B, the method based on convolution kernels was used to identify the PS, and the white circle indicates the point that was identified with this technique.

Fig. 3D illustrates the phase map of **Fig. 3**A, calculated using a time delay embedding with a delay of 150 ms (similar to that illustrated in **Fig. 2**C). Although the overall phase pattern seems to be similar to **Fig. 3**B, there are 2 important differences. First, the PS at the center is identified as anticlockwise, and this is denoted by the use of the square rather than a circle. Second, an additional pair of PS (1 clockwise and 1 anticlockwise) is identified toward the top of the phase map. Neither of these features is consistent with subsequent snapshots of voltage, where there is clockwise rotation and no wave break toward the top of the panel (see **Fig. 3**C). Thus, in this example a poor choice of the time delay parameter has resulted in errors in the phase map, and hence incorrect identification of PS.

PHASE MAPPING FOR VENTRICULAR ARRHYTHMIAS

Experimental studies of reentry in the ventricles of animal hearts have used optical mapping and phase analysis to establish reentry as an important mechanism for sustaining VF in the rabbit heart,[32] identify and track PS in the pig heart,[33] examine

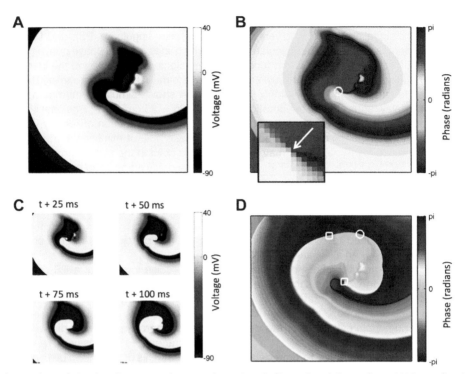

Fig. 3. (*A*) Snapshot of simulated transmembrane voltage in a 2-dimensional tissue sheet 1000 ms after initiation of reentry in a computational model of human ventricular tissue.[25] (*B*) Corresponding snapshot of phase angle calculated with time delay embedding and a delay of 20 ms (as shown in **Fig. 2B**). White circle denotes a clockwise phase singularity. Inset shows magnified view of the center of the plot with an arrow locating the phase singularity. (*C*) Subsequent snapshots of membrane voltage at 1025, 1050, 1075, and 1100 ms showing clockwise rotation. (*D*) Snapshot of phase calculated with time delay embedding and a delay of 150 ms (as shown in **Fig. 2C**). Squares indicate anticlockwise phase singularities and the circle indicates clockwise phase singularity.

the potential colocation of PS and anatomic features in rabbit hearts,[34] and examine the distribution of PS during VF with tissue heterogeneity in pig hearts.[35] The combination of optical mapping and phase analysis has thus become a well-established technique for this kind of experimental investigation.

Studies of VF in the human heart are much more difficult. Nevertheless, electrical mapping of fibrillation in the isolated myopathic human heart[36–38] and in the in situ human heart[5,39–41] has been combined with phase analysis to characterize reentry dynamics in the human heart during VF. A significant challenge in these investigations has been the use of electrodes with a spacing of around 1 cm. Earlier studies in the human heart using high-density electrical mapping established that VF was characterized by large wavefronts,[4] and so interpolation of electrogram voltages has been performed before phase analysis.[5,15] The potential impact of interpolation techniques on phase calculations and PS identification remains to be properly established.

Unipolar electrograms recorded during VF in the human heart are suitable for phase analysis,

provided that an appropriate embedding technique is used. **Fig. 4** shows an example from data recorded from the epicardial surface during VF initiated by burst pacing in patients undergoing cardiac surgery with cardiopulmonary bypass.[40] **Fig. 4A** shows a small extract of unipolar electrograms recorded from a single contact electrode. **Fig. 4B** shows the state-space representation when the time delay embedding is used with a delay of 60 ms, which was derived from the first minimum of the autocorrelation function. The origin is not at the center of the phase trajectories, and so phase would be incorrectly calculated using this approach. **Fig. 4C** shows the improvement in the phase trajectory obtained with the Hilbert transform. **Fig. 4D** shows a snapshot 1.8 s after initiation of VF of the epicardial electrogram voltage field, which has been interpolated from 256 electrodes over the entire ventricular epicardial surface as described elsewhere.[5] **Fig. 4E** shows the result of transforming the interpolated data into phase using the Hilbert transform. The 3 epicardial PS are shown as gray spheres, and wavefronts (lines of zero phase) are shown as black curves.[5]

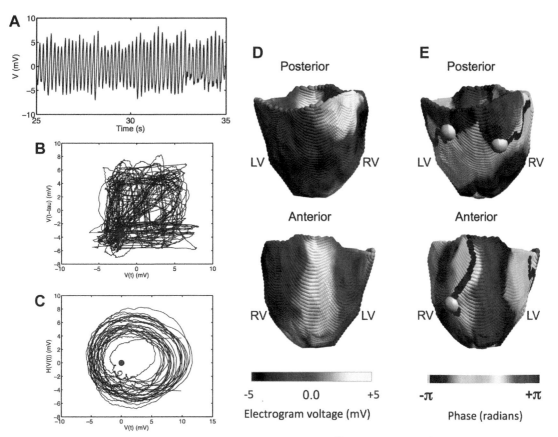

Fig. 4. Phase analysis of ventricular fibrillation in the human heart.[40] (A) Time series of electrogram voltage recorded from an epicardial electrode. (B) State-space representation of the time series using time delay embedding with a delay of 60 ms. Red circle indicates origin at (0,0). (C) State-space representation of the time series using the Hilbert transform as state variable on the vertical axis. (D) Snapshot of electrogram voltage interpolated over the ventricular epicardial surface, 1.8 s after initiation of VF. (E) Corresponding phase map calculated using the Hilbert transform. Gray spheres indicate phase singularities, and black lines wavefronts, which are lines of zero phase. LV, left ventricle; RV, right ventricle.

PHASE MAPPING FOR ATRIAL ARRHYTHMIAS

Contact electrograms recorded during AF possess sharper deflections than those recorded during VF. As a consequence, it is difficult to obtain a clear trajectory in state space when the raw electrogram is used as one of the state variables. This is illustrated clearly in a recent publication,[42] which describes a method to recompose the atrial electrogram as a sum of sine waves, where a single smooth deflection corresponds with each atrial activation in the raw signal. A similar approach has been used in other studies, where the atrial electrogram is used to reconstruct a sequence of monophasic action potentials.[43–45]

The noninvasive study of AF activation sequences in the human heart based on estimating epicardial potentials and electrograms from recordings taken using body surface electrodes is a recent development. This approach has been evaluated using simultaneous body surface and intra-atrial mapping,[10] and has been deployed with phase mapping for the quantitative analysis of reentry and focal activity during AF in the human heart.[11,46]

Both of these developments are significant because the results of recent studies indicate that directing ablation toward areas where reentry tends to occur may be effective in abolishing AF. Important questions remain about the mechanisms that are involved, but nevertheless it is likely that phase analysis will have a significant role in shaping interventions in the future, and it will be crucial to ensure that implementation is done carefully.

RECOMMENDATIONS

We recommend that studies in which phase analysis is to be used for the study of reentry in the human heart should take account of the following points when developing a processing pipeline.

- Preprocess signals to ensure that each cycle of activation and recovery is represented as a complete rotation around the origin in state-space. This will include:
  - Rejection of any signals that are noisy, for example, because of high contact impedance.
  - High-pass filtering to remove baseline movement, and low-pass filtering to remove powerline interference. For fibrillation in the human heart, the frequency range of interest is between 1 and 15 Hz.
  - Recomposition of electrograms recorded during AF as a sum of sine waves,[42] or piecewise detrending of electrograms recorded during VF.[29,31]
- Use the Hilbert transform[31] to calculate the second state-space variable W.
- Calculate the phase using the *atan2* function.
- Identify the phase singularities using convolution kernels.[27]

DISCUSSION

Phase mapping is a powerful approach for the analysis of cardiac arrhythmias when applied to signals recorded, either from electrode arrays or from optical mapping with voltage-sensitive fluorescent dyes. Several recent studies have used phase analysis for investigating mechanisms of AF and VF in the human heart. There is promise that the use of phase analysis may guide successful intervention.

A particular strength of phase analysis is that it enables PS to be identified, and thus the intricate patterns of electrical activation that sustain fibrillation can be characterized. The simplest approach is to estimate the complexity of fibrillation by counting the number of PS. A development of this idea is to track PS,[33] so that their locations and lifetimes can be quantified. In the experimental setting, these studies have shown that anatomic[34] or functional[35] heterogeneities can lead to clustering of PS. Moreover, the distribution of PS lifetimes is exponential,[32,33] which means that short-lived wavebreaks can be distinguished from longer lived rotors that play a more significant role in sustaining fibrillation.[47] This is potentially important for the study of mechanisms of AF.

Other techniques in addition to phase analysis have been used to examine and quantify reentrant activity during fibrillation. Automated identification and tracking of wavefronts during VF enables reentry to be identified and the provenance of

each wavefront to be established.[48] More recent studies of AF have tracked activation sequences using techniques derived from neuroscience,[49] and examined the similarity of deflections at each electrode.[50–52] Fusion of these approaches with phase mapping in the future may provide a more robust way to examine activation during AF, and so to guide intervention.

Despite these advantages, there are potential pitfalls in the different ways that phase is calculated from raw signals. Given the potential of phase analysis to guide clinical intervention, it is important that these issues are not overlooked. It is, therefore, suggested that the recommendations listed herein be carefully considered when using phase analysis of electrograms.

SUMMARY

Models of atrial cell and tissue electrophysiology combined with a detailed representation of human atrial anatomy have yielded insights into the electrophysiologic mechanisms that initiate and sustain both AF and VF.[53] Using such models as tools to validate phase mapping and to develop new techniques for quantifying the complexity of activation sequences during AF and VF is likely to be a fruitful area of future research.

ACKNOWLEDGMENTS

The data shown in **Fig. 4** were collected as part of a study of VF in the human heart,[40] with our colleagues Dr Chris Bradley, Professor Peter Taggart, Mr Martin Hayward, and Professor David Paterson.

REFERENCES

1. Rogers JM, Ideker RE. Fibrillating myocardium. Rabbit warren or beehive. Circulation 2000;86: 369–70.
2. Vaquero M, Calvo D, Jalife J. Cardiac fibrillation: from ion channels to rotors in the human heart. Heart Rhythm 2008;5(6):872–9.
3. Pandit SV, Jalife J. Rotors and the dynamics of cardiac fibrillation. Circ Res 2013;112(5):849–62.
4. Nanthakumar K, Walcott GP, Melnick S, et al. Epicardial organization of human ventricular fibrillation. Heart Rhythm 2004;1:14–23.
5. Nash MP, Mourad A, Clayton RH, et al. Evidence for multiple mechanisms in human ventricular fibrillation. Circulation 2006;114:536–42.
6. Narayan SM, Krummen DE, Enyeart MW, et al. Computational mapping identifies localized mechanisms for ablation of atrial fibrillation. PLoS One 2012;7:e46034.

7. Witkowski FX, Leon LJ, Penkoske PA, et al. Spatio-temporal evolution of ventricular fibrillation. Nature 1998;392:78–82.

8. Efimov IR, Nikolski VP, Salama G. Optical imaging of the heart. Circ Res 2004;286:H2183–94.

9. Laughner JI, Ng FS, Sulkin MS, et al. Processing and analysis of cardiac optical mapping data obtained with potentiometric dyes. Am J Physiol Heart Circ Physiol 2012;303:H753–65.

10. Cuculich PS, Wang Y, Lindsay BD, et al. Noninvasive characterization of epicardial activation in humans with diverse atrial fibrillation patterns. Circulation 2010;122:1364–72.

11. Haissaguerre M, Hocini M, Denis A, et al. Driver domains in persistent atrial fibrillation. Circulation 2014;130:530–8.

12. Winfree AT. When time breaks down. The three dimensional dynamics of electrochemical waves and cardiac arrhythmias. Princeton (NJ): Princeton University Press; 1987. p. 339.

13. Gray R, Pertsov AM, Jalife J. Spatial and temporal organization during cardiac fibrillation. Nature 1998;392:75–8.

14. Pogwizd SM, Hoyt RH, Saffitz JE, et al. Reentrant and focal mechanisms underlying ventricular tachycardia in the human heart. Circulation 1992;86:1872–87.

15. Umapathy K, Nair K, Masse S, et al. Phase mapping of cardiac fibrillation. Circ Arrhythm Electrophysiol 2010;3:105–14.

16. Clayton RH, Zhuchkova E, Panfilov AV. Phase singularities and filaments: simplifying complexity in computational models of ventricular fibrillation. Prog Biophys Mol Biol 2006;90:378–98.

17. Allessie MA, Bonke F, Schopman F. Circus movement in rabbit atrial muscle as a mechanism of tachycardia. Circ Res 1973;33:54–62.

18. Allessie MA, Bonke FI, Schopman FJ. Circus movement in rabbit atrial muscle as a mechanism of tachycardia. III. The "leading circle" concept: a new model of circus movement in cardiac tissue without the involvement of an anatomical obstacle. Circ Res 1977;41:9–18.

19. Ideker RE, Frazier DW, Krassowska W, et al. Experimental evidence for autowaves in the heart. Ann N Y Acad Sci 1990;591:208–18.

20. Pogwizd SM, Corr PB. Mechanisms underlying the development of ventricular fibrillation during early myocardial ischaemia. Circ Res 1990;66:672–95.

21. Davidenko JM, Pertsov AM, Salomonsz R, et al. Stationary and drifting spiral waves of excitation in isolated cardiac muscle. Nature 1992;355:349–51.

22. Pertsov AM, Davidenko JM, Salomonsz R, et al. Spiral waves of excitation underlie reentrant activity in isolated cardiac muscle. Circ Res 1993;72:631–50.

23. Iyer A, Gray R. An experimentalist's approach to accurate localization of phase singularities during reentry. Ann Biomed Eng 2001;29:47–59.

24. Sambelashvilli A, Efimov IR. Dynamics of virtual electrode-induced scroll-wave reentry in a 3D bidomain model. Am J Physiol Heart Circ Physiol 2004;287:H1570–81.

25. Clayton RH, Nash MP, Bradley CP, et al. Experiment-model interaction for analysis of epicardial activation during human ventricular fibrillation with global myocardial ischaemia. Prog Biophys Mol Biol 2011;107:101–11.

26. Ten Tusscher KH, Panfilov AV. Alternans and spiral breakup in a human ventricular tissue model. Am J Physiol Heart Circ Physiol 2006;291:1088–100.

27. Bray MA, Wikswo JP. Use of topological charge to determine filament location and dynamics in a numerical model of scroll wave activity. IEEE Trans Biomed Eng 2002;49:1086–93.

28. Clayton RH. Vortex filament dynamics in computational models of ventricular fibrillation in the heart. Chaos 2008;18:43127.

29. Rogers JM. Combined phase singularity and wavefront analysis for optical maps of ventricular fibrillation. IEEE Trans Biomed Eng 2004;92:56–65.

30. Packard NH, Crutchfield JP, Farmer JD, et al. Geometry from a time series. Phys Rev Lett 1980;45:712–6.

31. Bray MA, Wikswo J. Considerations in phase plane analysis for nonstationary reentrant cardiac behavior. Phys Rev E Stat Nonlin Soft Matter Phys 2002;65:1–8.

32. Chen J, Mandapati R, Berenfeld O, et al. High-frequency periodic sources underlie ventricular fibrillation in the isolated rabbit heart. Circ Res 2000;86:86–93.

33. Kay MW, Walcott GP, Gladden JD, et al. Lifetimes of epicardial rotors in panoramic optical maps of fibrillating swine ventricles. Am J Physiol Heart Circ Physiol 2006;291:H1935–41.

34. Valderrábano M, Chen P, Lin S. Spatial distribution of phase singularities in ventricular fibrillation. Circulation 2003;108:354–9.

35. Zaitsev AV, Guha PK, Sarmast F, et al. Wavebreak formation during ventricular fibrillation in the isolated, regionally ischemic pig heart. Circ Res 2003;92:546–53.

36. Masse S, Downar E, Chauhan V, et al. Ventricular fibrillation in myopathic human hearts: mechanistic insights from in vivo global endocardial and epicardial mapping. Am J Physiol Heart Circ Physiol 2007;292:H2589–97.

37. Farid T, Nair K, Masse S, et al. Role of KATP channels in the maintenance of ventricular fibrillation in cardiomyopathic human hearts. Circ Res 2011;109:1309–18.

38. Umapathy K, Massé S, Sevaptsidis E, et al. Spatiotemporal frequency analysis of ventricular fibrillation in explanted human hearts. IEEE Trans Biomed Eng 2009;56:328–35.

39. Ten Tusscher KH, Mourad A, Nash MP, et al. Organization of ventricular fibrillation in the human heart: experiments and models. Exp Physiol 2009;94:553–62.

40. Bradley CP, Clayton RH, Nash MP, et al. Human ventricular fibrillation during global ischemia and reperfusion: paradoxical changes in activation rate and wavefront complexity. Circ Arrhythm Electrophysiol 2011;4:684–91.

41. Krummen DE, Hayase J, Morris DJ, et al. Rotor stability separates sustained ventricular fibrillation from self-terminating episodes in humans. J Am Coll Cardiol 2014;63:2712–21.

42. Kuklik P, Zeemering S, Maesen B, et al. Reconstruction of instantaneous phase of unipolar atrial contact electrogram using a concept of sinusoidal recomposition and Hilbert transform. IEEE Trans Biomed Eng 2015. [Epub ahead of print].

43. Narayan SM, Krummen DE, Shivkumar K, et al. Treatment of atrial fibrillation by the ablation of localized sources: CONFIRM (Conventional Ablation for Atrial Fibrillation with or without Focal Impulse and Rotor Modulation) trial. J Am Coll Cardiol 2012;60:628–36.

44. Narayan SM, Krummen DE, Rappel WJ. Clinical mapping approach to diagnose electrical rotors and focal impulse sources for human atrial fibrillation. J Cardiovasc Electrophysiol 2012;23:447–54.

45. Narayan S, Rappel WJ. System for analysis of complex rhythm disorders. 2014; Patent application US 20140228696 A1.

46. Haissaguerre M, Hocini M, Shah AJ, et al. Noninvasive panoramic mapping of human atrial fibrillation mechanisms: a feasibility report. J Cardiovasc Electrophysiol 2013;24:711–7.

47. Rogers JM, Walcott GP, Gladden J, et al. Panoramic optical mapping reveals continuous epicardial reentry during ventricular fibrillation in the isolated swine heart. Biophys J 2007;92:1090–5.

48. Rogers JM, Usui M, KenKnight BH, et al. A quantitative framework for analyzing epicardial activation patterns during ventricular fibrillation. Ann Biomed Eng 1997;25:749–60.

49. Richter U, Faes L, Ravelli F, et al. Propagation pattern analysis during atrial fibrillation based on sparse modeling. IEEE Trans Biomed Eng 2012;59:1319–28.

50. Ravelli F, Masè M. Computational mapping in atrial fibrillation: how the integration of signal-derived maps may guide the localization of critical sources. Europace 2014;16:714–23.

51. Faes L, Nollo G, Antolini R, et al. A method for quantifying atrial fibrillation organization based on wave-morphology similarity. IEEE Trans Biomed Eng 2002;49:1504–13.

52. Ravelli F, Faes L, Sandrini L, et al. Wave similarity mapping shows the spatiotemporal distribution of fibrillatory wave complexity in the human right atrium during paroxysmal and chronic atrial fibrillation. J Cardiovasc Electrophysiol 2005;16:1071–6.

53. Trayanova NA, O'Hara T, Bayer JD, et al. Computational cardiology: how computer simulations could be used to develop new therapies and advance existing ones. Europace 2012;14:v82–9.

Frontiers in Noninvasive Cardiac Mapping
Rotors in Atrial Fibrillation-Body Surface Frequency-Phase Mapping

CrossMark

Felipe Atienza, MD[a], Andreu M. Climent, PhD[a],
María S. Guillem, PhD[b], Omer Berenfeld, PhD, FHRS[c],*

KEYWORDS

- Atrial fibrillation • Body surface mapping • Rotors • Dominant frequency • Fourier transform
- Phase mapping

KEY POINTS

- Atrial fibrillation (AF) maintenance in experiments and certain groups of patients depends on localized reentrant sources with fibrillatory conduction to the remainder of the atria.
- AF can be eliminated by directly ablating AF-driving sources or "rotors" that exhibit high-frequency, periodic activity.
- The RADAR-AF randomized clinical trial demonstrated that in paroxysmal AF patients, selective ablation of highest frequency sites responsible for AF maintenance is as effective as circumferential pulmonary vein isolation, and decreased ablation risks.
- Body surface potential map (BSPM) dominant frequency estimation allows the global identification of high-frequency sources driving AF before and during the electrophysiology laboratory procedure for ablation.
- Phase maps of highest dominant frequency–filtered BSPM recordings allow prior and real-time noninvasive localization of atrial reentries during AF, enabling further physiologically based rationale for personalized AF ablation procedures.

 Videos of rotor trajectories accompany this article at http://www.cardiacep.theclinics.com/

Sources of funding: Study supported in part by the Spanish Society of Cardiology (Becas Investigación Clínica 2009); the Universitat Politècnica de València through its research initiative program; the Generalitat Valenciana Grants (ACIF/2013/021); the Ministerio de Economia y Competividad, Red RIC; the Centro Nacional de Investigaciones Cardiovasculares (proyecto CNIC-13); the Coulter Foundation from the Biomedical Engineering Department (University of Michigan); the Gelman Award from the Cardiovascular Division (University of Michigan); the National Heart, Lung, and Blood Institute grants (P01-HL039707, P01-HL087226 and R01-HL118304), and the Leducq Foundation.
Conflicts of interest: Felipe Atienza, MD served on the advisory board of Medtronic and has received research funding from St. Jude Medical Spain. Omer Berenfeld, PhD, FHRSc received research support from Medtronic and St. Jude Medical. He is a co-founder, share-holder and Scientific Officer of Rhythm Solutions, Inc. Other authors have no conflicts to report. None of the companies disclosed here financed the research described in this article.
[a] Cardiology Department, Hospital General Universitario Gregorio Marañón, Calle Doctor Esquerdo 46, Madrid 28009, Spain; [b] Bio-ITACA, Universitat Politècnica de València, Camino de Vera s/n, Valencia 46022, Spain; [c] Center for Arrhythmia Research, Department of Internal Medicine, University of Michigan, 2800 Plymouth Road, Ann Arbor, MI 48109, USA
* Corresponding author.
E-mail address: oberen@umich.edu

Card Electrophysiol Clin 7 (2015) 59–69
http://dx.doi.org/10.1016/j.ccep.2014.11.002

INTRODUCTION

Atrial fibrillation (AF) is the most common arrhythmia seen in clinical practice and is associated with increased risk of stroke, heart failure, and death.[1] Although antiarrhythmic drugs have limited efficacy, the demonstration of AF triggers in the atrial sleeves of the pulmonary veins (PVs) has led to a significant improvement in therapy.[2,3] Several ablative strategies have been developed with the objective of creating circumferential lesions around the PV ostia.[4] Empiric circumferential pulmonary vein isolation (CPVI) is effective in ~70 to 80% of patients with paroxysmal AF and has become therapy of choice for drug-refractory AF in these patients.[5] However, results still remain suboptimal because of the presence of non-PV sources maintaining AF.[4,6,7] Moreover, the success rate of CPVI in the more prevalent persistent and long-lasting AF populations is significantly lower and extensive substrate-based ablation strategies have been used with conflicting results.[8,9]

Experimental and clinical data from the authors' laboratory support the hypothesis that both acute and persistent AF in the sheep and some groups of human patients is not a random phenomenon. Studies analyzing the spatiotemporal organization of waves and dominant frequency (DF) in the isolated sheep heart demonstrate that AF maintenance in this model depends on localized reentrant sources in the left atrium (LA) and fibrillatory conduction in its periphery.[10–15] As a natural consequence of these studies, the authors translated the analysis on the organization of DF to human AF and found that AF reentrant sources are localized primarily to the PVs and LA posterior wall in the case of paroxysmal AF but elsewhere in the case of persistent AF.[16–20] Several of these observational studies showed that AF could be eliminated by directly ablating AF-driving sources or "rotors" that exhibit high-frequency, periodic activity, based on either electrogram (EGM) visual analysis, DF analysis, or panoramic endocardial mapping.[2,17–19,21–25] Recently, the first randomized clinical trial, RADAR-AF, demonstrated that, in paroxysmal AF patients selective ablation of sites responsible for AF maintenance is as effective as CPVI and decreased ablation risks.[26] These results demonstrate that an ablation procedure based on a more target-specific strategy aimed at eliminating high-frequency sites responsible for AF maintenance is efficacious and is safer than empirically isolating all the PVs.

Therefore, it would be arguably desirable to noninvasively identify the location of the sources responsible for AF maintenance before the procedure to design the ideal ablation strategy for each individual AF patient as well as to be able to perform a panoramic real-time localization of sources during the procedure.[27,28] Although the highest-frequency sources in paroxysmal AF are most commonly located in the junction of the LA with the PVs, they have also been identified elsewhere in the atria and may shift in time. Recent studies by the authors' group have shown that panoramic, global, atrial noninvasive frequency analysis is feasible in AF patients and may allow the identification of high-frequency sources before the arrival at the electrophysiology laboratory for ablation. Body surface map (BSPM) replicates the endocardial distribution of DFs and can identify small areas containing the high-frequency sources that result in fibrillatory conduction to the reminder of the atria and may decrease the time required for the search and elimination of the highest DF (HDF) site.[29] Moreover, the authors recently showed that phase maps of surface potentials during AF after HDF filtering allowed the observation of driving reentrant patterns ("rotors") with spatiotemporal stability for greater than 70% of the AF time.[30] Thus, as shown in the following sections, the ability of BSPM to detect sites driving AF may enable a noninvasive personalized diagnosis and treatment of patients with AF.

THE NONINVASIVE MAPPING SYSTEM

In the authors' studies, AF patients wore a custom-made, adjustable vest with 64 electrodes covering the entire torso surface (**Fig. 1**) during the ablation procedure.[17,29,30] The vest included recording electrodes on the anterior (N = 28), posterior (N = 34), and lateral sides (N = 2) of the torso. In addition, 3 limb leads were recorded and used to generate the Wilson terminal. The BSPM vest was placed before the catheterization and fastened anteriorly, allowing access to the patient's chest in case external electrical cardioversion was needed during the course of the study. Surface unipolar electrocardiographic recordings were obtained by using a commercial system for bio-potential measurements (Active Two, Biosemi, The Netherlands) at a sampling frequency of 2048 Hz and stored on hard disk for off-line analyses.[31] Ventricular activity was removed from the unipolar recordings before analysis numerically or by application of adenosine.[29]

SPECTRAL ANALYSIS OF BODY SURFACE POTENTIAL MAPPING

Previous studies have highlighted the major role of maximal DF (DFmax) sources in the maintenance of AF in animals and humans.[14,17,32] Arguably,

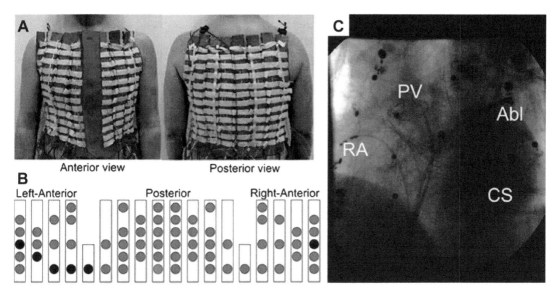

Fig. 1. The setup of the body surface recording electrodes. (*A*) Anterior and posterior views of the custom-made vest with 64 recording electrodes along vertical blue strips. (*B*) Schematic location of surface electrodes. Circles represent the location of recording electrodes. Electrodes representing the standard ECG precordial leads are denoted as black circles. (*C*) Radiographic image displaying the locations of the intracardiac recording catheters together with the surface leads. Abl, ablation catheter; CS, coronary sinus; PV, circular mapping at the right superior pulmonary vein. (*From* Guillem MS, Climent AM, Millet J, et al. Noninvasive localization of maximal frequency sites of atrial fibrillation by body surface potential mapping. Circ Arrhythm Electrophysiol 2013;6:295; with permission. Copyright © American Heart Association, Inc. All rights reserved.)

prior knowledge of which atrium harbors the DFmax source that maintains the arrhythmia may allow better planning of the ablation procedure and may accelerate the intracardiac localization of the HDF point and reduce ablation time. Thus, the authors explored the ability of the body surface DFs to capture the intracardiac DFmax.

Surface leads and simultaneously recorded intracardiac signals presented closely related spectral components. In **Fig. 2**, spectral analyses of data are presented from a representative patient in whom the presence of a distinct atrial site with high-frequency activity in the posterior LA could be determined noninvasively. In **Fig. 2**A, 3 representative EGMs illustrate the range of activation rates across the atria, with DFs ranging from 5.75 Hz in the right atrium (RA) to 7 Hz in the LA near the left superior pulmonary vein. Simultaneously recorded surface leads also showed different DFs at nearly the same frequency range found in the EGM recordings, as shown in **Fig. 2**B by 3 representative leads corresponding to the surface left, surface back (SB), and surface right regions. Surface DFs mostly correlated with the activation rate of nearest atrial tissue: the highest endocardial DF point was observed at the nearest point on the torso surface (central posterior) and the lowest activation rate of the RA was found at the nearest portion of the

surface electrocardiogram (ECG; right inferior). Intracardiac CARTO DF maps obtained before adenosine infusion and surface DF distributions obtained during adenosine infusion showed good correspondence (see **Fig. 2**C, D), but a direct comparison of frequencies from CARTO and surface maps was unattainable because of its sequential nature and because adenosine accelerates AF activation in humans.[18]

Fig. 3A, B displays difference maps obtained by subtracting DF values on the surface map from the intracardiac DFmax in patients from **Fig. 2** and another patient in which the DFmax resides in the RA. In each case, the white arrow points to the red-colored DFmax domain on the surface, which corresponds to the region with zero difference with the intracardiac DFmax. These examples demonstrate that the surface DFmax can accurately detect the value of the intracardiac DFmax value, regardless of whether the latter is localized to the LA or the RA. To further analyze the correspondence between intracardiac and surface AF frequencies in the RA and LA, the authors grouped the intracardiac DFmax values measured in the LA and RA and correlated them with the DFs of EGMs from matching portions on the body surface. These matching portions were defined as those in which the difference between the intracardiac DFmax in each atrium and the

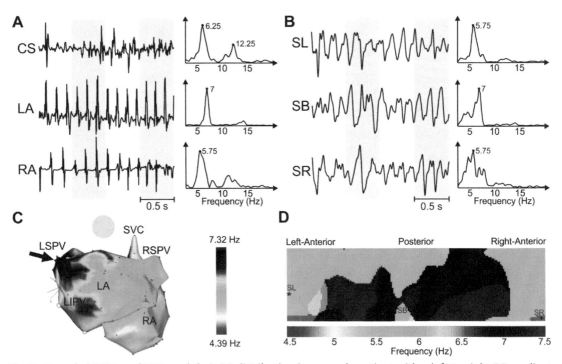

Fig. 2. Recorded EGMs and ECGs and their DF distribution in a sample patient with a left-to-right DF gradient. (*A*) Three examples of EGMs recorded at different atrial sites and their corresponding power spectra. (*B*) Selected surface BSPM leads: surface left (SL), surface back (SB), and surface right (SR), and their corresponding power spectra. (*C*) Intracardiac DF map. Black arrow points to the LA region with HDF at the left superior pulmonary vein (LSPV). (*D*) DF map on the torso surface with superimposed locations of electrodes from (*B*). CS, coronary sinus; LIPV, left inferior pulmonary vein; RSPV, right superior pulmonary vein; SVC, superior vena cava. (*Adapted from* Guillem MS, Climent AM, Millet J, et al. Noninvasive localization of maximal frequency sites of atrial fibrillation by body surface potential mapping. Circ Arrhythm Electrophysiol 2013;6:296; with permission. Copyright © American Heart Association, Inc. All rights reserved.)

surface DFmax was 0.5 Hz or less. **Fig. 3**C, D shows that when the entire patient population under study was included, there was a good correspondence between maximum DFs found in each atrial chamber and right and left matching portions of the body surface, respectively. The correlation between right surface leads and right intracardiac EGMs was 0.96, whereas correlation for left leads with left intracardiac EGMs was 0.92 (see **Fig. 3**E, F). The attempted correlation of surface leads with EGMs of the opposed atrial chamber yielded much lower correlation values (RA body surface leads vs intracardiac LA EGMs, 0.26; one-tailed *t* test after Fisher r-to-z transform: *P*<.0001 vs *r* = 0.96; left body surface leads vs intracardiac RA EGMs, 0.46; *P* = .0052 vs *r* = 0.92).

Such a strong, side-specific correspondence of frequencies enabled reliable determination of atrial frequency gradients noninvasively.[29] The DF gradients on the 64 electrodes of the BSPM showed a good correlation with the DF gradients obtained by the simultaneous intracardiac EGMs (correlation

coefficient = 0.93). On the other hand, surface frequency gradients estimated by the standard precordial ECG leads yielded a poor correspondence with gradients estimated from the intracardiac EGMs, with a correlation coefficient equal to 0.41 when considering all 6 standard leads, or equal to 0.51 when considering only V1 and V6 (*P* = .0051 when compared with the correlation of the full BSPM DF gradients).[27,29]

To predict the ability of the BSPM to detect intracardiac LA-to-RA DF gradients, the authors classified patients with a LA-RA gradient in DF (maximal right and left values differ by more than 0.5 Hz) versus without LA-RA gradient otherwise. Overall, the sensitivity of the BSPM to capture intracardiac EGMs as having LA-RA gradient in DF was 75%, but the specificity of the BSPM in capturing those gradients was 100%. The sensitivity and specificity of the standard ECG leads V1 and V6 in detecting a LA-to-RA DF gradient were 67% and 50%, respectively. Although the BSPM was able to identify most, but not all, intracardiac DF gradients, each DF gradient identified

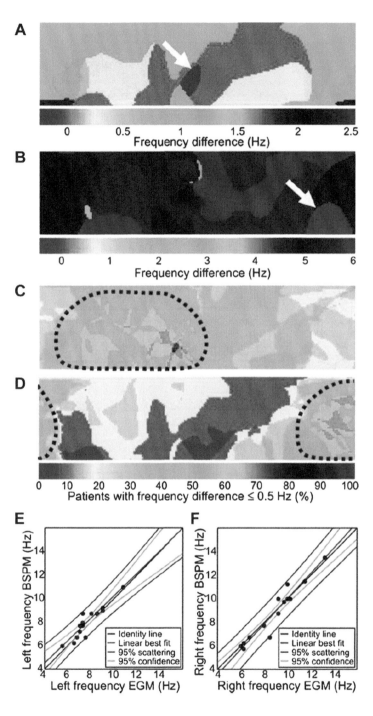

Fig. 3. Correspondence between intracardiac and surface DFs. (*A, B*) Differences between maximum intracardiac EGM DF and local surface DF represented in a color scale for 2 different patients. The red color domain on the surface (*white arrows*) represents the region with zero difference between the intracardiac and surface DFs. (*A*) Patient from **Fig. 2** with a left-to-right DF gradient. (*B*) Patient with a right-to-left DF gradient. (*C, D*) Summary maps showing the percentage of patients with the surface DFs less than 0.5 Hz different than the maximal left (*C*) and maximal right (*D*) intracardiac DFs. Areas outlined by the dashed curves represent the portion of the torso with a best correspondence with left and right EGMs. (*E*) Correlation plot showing HDFs found in left EGMs versus HDFs found on the left portion of the torso. (*F*) Correlation plot showing HDFs found in right EGMs versus HDFs found on the right portion of the torso. (*From* Guillem MS, Climent AM, Millet J, et al. Noninvasive localization of maximal frequency sites of atrial fibrillation by body surface potential mapping. Circ Arrhythm Electrophysiol 2013;6: 298; with permission. Copyright © American Heart Association, Inc. All rights reserved.)

by the BSPM was a true gradient as determined by the intracardiac recordings. Standard ECG leads, however, allowed the detection of a lower proportion of patients with LA-to-RA DF gradients as compared with all BSPM leads and also mistakenly identified LA-RA DF gradients that were not confirmed in the EGM recordings.

SURFACE MAPPING OF ATRIAL PATTERNS OF ACTIVITY DURING ATRIAL FIBRILLATION

Surface phase maps of the unipolar voltage time series recorded during AF show unstable patterns, as can be appreciated by the transient singularity points (SPs) seen in the maps from a sample patient presented in the left panel of **Fig. 4**A.[30]

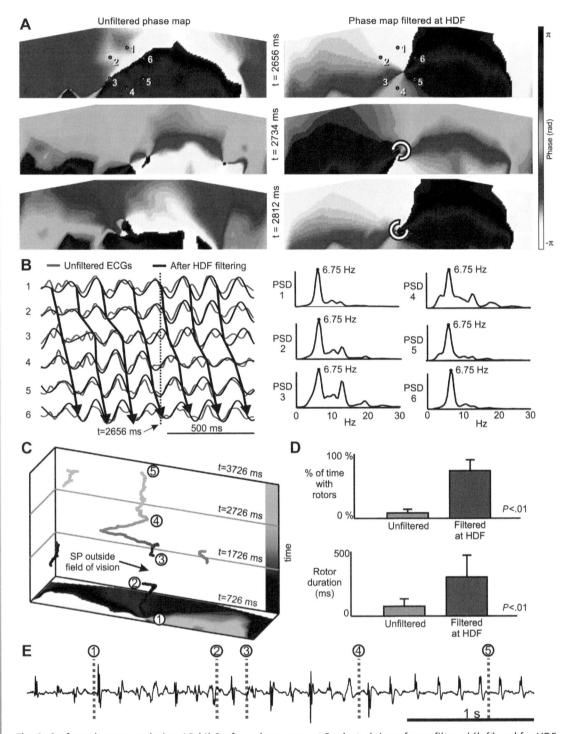

Fig. 4. Surface phase maps during AF. (*A*) Surface phase maps at 3 selected times for unfiltered (*left*) and for HDF-filtered (*right*) surface potentials. (*B*) ECGs at positions 1 to 6 marked in (*A*) before and after HDF filtering and power spectral density (PSD) for unfiltered ECGs. Time marker at 2656 ms corresponds to the top map in the HDF-filtered data in (*A*). (*C*) PSs trajectories on the torso surface during a 3-second-long AF. (*D*) Percentage of time with rotors (*top*) and rotor duration (*bottom*) in surface phase maps from unfiltered and HDF-filtered surface potentials over the entire cohort. (*E*) EGM recorded at the HDF site in the atria (RSPV) simultaneously with the surface recordings. (*From* Rodrigo M, Guillem MS, Climent AM, et al. Body surface localization of left and right atrial high-frequency rotors in atrial fibrillation patients: a clinical-computational study. Heart Rhythm 2014;11(9):1586; with permission.)

Long-lasting SPs were rarely observed during AF without band-pass filtering, and those observed tended to drift erratically large distances in a short time. However, after band-pass filtering of the potential signal around the HDF (6.8 Hz), surface phase maps showed more stable SPs for the same AF episode (see **Fig. 4**A, *right panel*). In **Fig. 4**B, the arrows connecting sequential activations in ECGs recorded around the SP in **Fig. 4**A show a clear reentrant pattern, which following HDF filtering transformed into long-lasting rotational patterns with stable SPs. Considering data from all patients, stable SPs were found in unfiltered AF signals during 8.3 ± 5.7% of the time versus 73.1 ± 16.8% following HDF-filtered signals (P<.01). The average SPs' duration concomitantly increased following the HDF filtering (160 ± 43 vs 342 ± 138 ms, P<.01). At an average HDF of 9.2 ± 2.3 (BSPM) or 9.3 ± 2.0 (EGM) Hz, the latter corresponds to an average of 2.9 ± 0.7 continuous rotations per SP observed in the authors' cohort of 14 patients.[30] Many observed SPs drift and appear or disappear on the borders of the surface mapped area, or in the beginning and end of the periods analyzed; thus, this average number of rotations represents a lower limit for their lifespan. Indeed, **Fig. 4**C and Video 1 (available online at http://www.cardiacep.theclinics.com/) show a rotor in the middle of the mapped area at the beginning of the period analyzed that after about 1400 ms disappears at the lower boundary of the area. After a period of fuzzy SP behavior in the posterior torso (see Video 1) for about 330 ms, an SP appears and remains in the mapped area for the rest of the analyzed period. This case shows that the actual lifespan of rotors could be longer than the conservative average lifespan the authors calculate. Further evidence of atrial rotor drifting is provided by the simultaneous EGM recorded at the HDF site (see **Fig. 4**E), which is unstable in intervals 1 to 4 and monomorphic at intervals 4 to 5, which is consistent with the observed drifting on the torso surface.

SIMULATIONS TO UNDERSTAND HIGHEST DOMINANT FREQUENCY BAND-PASS FILTERING OF ATRIAL FIBRILLATION PATTERNS

The finding that the dynamics of the body surface SPs dramatically depends on the HDF filtering raises questions regarding the phase maps interpretation. Unfortunately, the ability to collect electrical data simultaneously in the atria and inside the torso volume and surface to make inferences between atrial activity and its manifestation on the body surface is limited, leading us to rely on computer simulations for guidance.

In **Fig. 5**, a simulation with an LA–RA atrial model and the multispheres torso model is depicted. In this model, there is a single functional rotor in the LA hemisphere turning at 7.2 Hz, while the RA hemisphere is passively activated at lower a frequency (3.9 Hz). **Fig. 2**A shows the phase maps of 3 concentric layers between the epicardium (*left*) and the torso surface (*right*) at various times. The phase maps become smoother toward the torso surface, reflecting the low-pass filter effect of the passive torso volume on the extracellular potentials. In the epicardial layer, there is one stable SP at the location of the functional rotor (LA) that appears at similar positions in the outer layers, and another SP at the less stable wave-break location at the interface between the faster LA and the slower RA. Azimuth and elevation of SPs detected on the surface are not preserved across layers, so the filament arising from the LA rotor exhibits a deflection in its trajectory to the torso. The deflection angle of the filaments before HDF filtering is not stationary over time and, instead, the filament trajectory describes a cone. However, **Fig. 5**B shows that HDF filtering significantly reduces the filaments' deflection and stabilizes them to follow a straight path from the epicardium to the surface. The simulations suggested that SPs arising at the interface between LA and RA as a consequence of abrupt changes in propagation direction that reached the outermost layer disappear after HDF filtering because their activation frequencies did not match with the HDF.[30] In addition, the authors notice that a mirror filament appears with opposite direction and chirality as compared with the true rotor originating at the SP on the LA epicardium. Indeed, following the attenuation of RA activation frequencies, potentials on the RA hemisphere are caused by the rotating electrical activity on the LA and observed from a contralateral point of view.

THE TORSO AS A LOW-PASS FILTER FOR ROTOR ACTIVITY

The authors further explored the behavior of filaments under more complex wave patterns resulting from a 50% LA area and 50% fibrotic area model.[30] In this case, epicardial activity consists of a LA rotor with a stable SP and a highly disorganized activity with several unstable SPs in the fibrotic area. Most of the filaments originate at SPs involving a small piece of fibrotic tissue and not at the driving rotor. In that case, the torso volume conductor stabilizes filaments and eliminates all but a single filaments' pair reaching

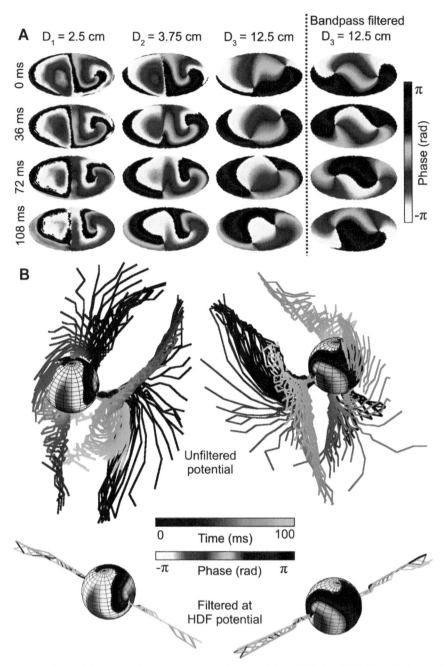

Fig. 5. Epicardial and transition to surface phase maps during AF in a 50% LA–50% RA atrial model. (*A*) Phase maps at 4 time instants (*top to bottom*) in 3 concentric layers at increasing distances from the epicardium (*left to right*) and after HDF filtering of surface potentials. (*B*) Phase map of epicardial sphere and temporal distribution of filaments for unfiltered potentials and for HDF-filtered potentials. (*Adapted from* Rodrigo M, Guillem MS, Climent AM, et al. Body surface localization of left and right atrial high-frequency rotors in atrial fibrillation patients: a clinical-computational study. Heart Rhythm 2014;11(9):1587; with permission.)

the surface. The simulations clearly show that filaments are continuous and do not vanish inside the passive volume conductor; rather, a filament does not reach the surface once it is joining its counter-rotating neighbor. Overall, that mutual cancellation of filament pairs reduces the average number of SPs at increasing distances from the epicardium.

However, as shown in **Fig. 5**, only one of the SPs on the body surface is a "true" SP corresponding to a driving rotor, and others are termed "mirror" SPs because they appear following the extinction of an SP at the LA-RA interface, as shown in **Fig. 5**, or extinction of SPs in fibrotic area, with an extension of the stable LA rotor filament to the contralateral aspect of the torso.[30] Indeed, the discrimination between true and mirror SPs can be performed based on the spectral properties of surface recordings. Although on the phase map these SPs seem undistinguishable, the spectral power at the HDF, the rotor frequency band, should be maximal only at "true" SPs.[30]

REGIONS OF BODY SURFACE ROTATIONAL ACTIVITY IN HUMAN ATRIAL FIBRILLATION (FILAMENTS)

True SPs detected, defined as those with at least 60% of their spectral content at the HDF band, tended to concentrate at certain torso areas. In **Fig. 6**A, the trajectory of a surface SP that drifted for 2 seconds on the posterior torso of a patient following LA-HDF filtering (band-pass filtering at the HDF found in simultaneous left intracardiac EGMs recordings) is depicted (see Video 1). In **Fig. 6**B, the trajectory of an SP that drifted during 500 ms on the right anterior torso in another patient after RA-HDF filtering is shown (see

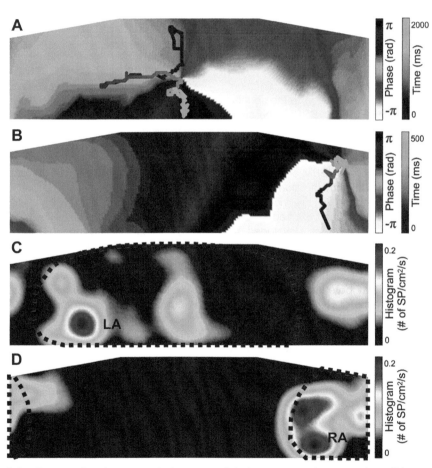

Fig. 6. Spatial distribution of surface rotors in human AF. (*A*) Phase map and rotor tracking (*blue scale*) after LA-HDF filtering in an LA-fastest patient. (*B*) Phase map and rotor tracking (*blue scale*) after RA-HDF filtering in an RA-fastest patient. (*C*) Histogram of the rotor position for all rotors detected in patients with an interatrial DF gradient after LA-HDF filtering. LA-detected region is outlined with a dotted line. (*D*) Histogram of the rotor position for all rotors detected in patients with an interatrial DF gradient after RA-HDF filtering. RA-detected region is outlined with a dotted line. (*From* Rodrigo M, Guillem MS, Climent AM, et al. Body surface localization of left and right atrial high-frequency rotors in atrial fibrillation patients: a clinical-computational study. Heart Rhythm 2014;11(9):1589; with permission.)

Video 2, available online at http://www.cardia-cep.theclinics.com/). In **Fig. 6**C, the 2-dimensional histogram of "true" SP locations after LA-HDF filtering in patients with an interatrial DF gradient greater than 1 Hz (n = 10) shows a predominant location of SPs on the posterior torso. The 2-dimensional histogram of "true" SP locations after RA-HDF filtering in patients with interatrial DF gradient shows a predominant localization on the right anterior torso (see **Fig. 6**D). The locations of the maximal numbers of true LA or RA SPs (dark red regions) are shown in **Fig. 6**C, D to reside well within the areas demarcated by the HDFs originating at either the LA or the RA, respectively, based on the previous surface-atrial DF distribution correlation study.[29]

SUMMARY AND CLINICAL IMPLICATIONS

Global atrial noninvasive frequency analysis is feasible in AF patients and may allow the identification of high-frequency sources before the arrival at the electrophysiology laboratory for ablation. Importantly, the authors' results led to the conclusion that, unlike high-resolution BSPM, the standard precordial ECG leads alone are not a useful tool when attempting to localize the site of DFmax sites responsible for AF maintenance.

The clinical-computational BSPM study on patterns of activity suggests that the body surface data on wave-breaks during AF are incomplete, but it contains features that can be linked to reentrant drivers of AF. The authors developed an approach whereby a narrow band-pass filtering allows selection of the electrical activity projected on the torso at the HDF, which stabilizes the projection of rotors that potentially drive AF on the surface. Phase maps of HDF-filtered surface ECG recordings may allow the noninvasive localization of atrial reentries during AF, enabling further physiologically based rationale for considering the constraints of the inverse solutions.

Thus, the authors' approach of a full panoramic BSPM procedure may help in planning and performing ablation procedures, decreasing the amount of time required for the search of AF drivers. The approach could arguably be used in patient selection because patients without interchamber DF gradient or clear localized drivers have lower ablation success rates.[17] In addition, a priori knowledge of the chamber responsible for the maintenance of the arrhythmia in those patients presenting a DF gradient may help in planning and performing the ablation procedure, decreasing the time required for the search, and eliminating drivers and/or the HDF site.

VIDEOS

Videos related to this article can be found online at http://dx.doi.org/10.1016/j.ccep.2014.11.002.

REFERENCES

1. Wann LS, Curtis AB, January CT, et al. Members AATF. 2011 ACCF/AHA/HRS focused update on the management of patients with atrial fibrillation (updating the 2006 guideline): a report of the American College of Cardiology Foundation/American Heart Association task force on practice guidelines. Circulation 2011;123:104–23.
2. Dobrev D, Nattel S. New antiarrhythmic drugs for treatment of atrial fibrillation. Lancet 2010;375: 1212–23.
3. Haissaguerre M, Jais P, Shah DC, et al. Spontaneous initiation of atrial fibrillation by ectopic beats originating in the pulmonary veins. N Engl J Med 1998;339:659–66.
4. Calkins H, Kuck KH, Cappato R, et al. 2012 HRS/EHRA/ECAS Expert Consensus Statement on Catheter and Surgical Ablation of Atrial Fibrillation: recommendations for patient selection, procedural techniques, patient management and follow-up, definitions, endpoints, and research trial design. Europace 2012;14:528–606.
5. Pappone C, Oreto G, Rosanio S, et al. Atrial electroanatomic remodeling after circumferential radiofrequency pulmonary vein ablation - efficacy of an anatomic approach in a large cohort of patients with atrial fibrillation. Circulation 2001;104:2539–44.
6. Lin YJ, Tai CT, Kao T, et al. Frequency analysis in different types of paroxysmal atrial fibrillation. J Am Coll Cardiol 2006;47:1401–7.
7. Lin WS, Tai CT, Hsieh MH, et al. Catheter ablation of paroxysmal atrial fibrillation initiated by non-pulmonary vein ectopy. Circulation 2003;107:3176–83.
8. Haissaguerre M, Sanders P, Hocini M, et al. Catheter ablation of long-lasting persistent atrial fibrillation: critical structures for termination. J Cardiovasc Electrophysiol 2005;16:1125–37.
9. Weerasooriya R, Khairy P, Litalien J, et al. Catheter ablation for atrial fibrillation: are results maintained at 5 years of follow-up? J Am Coll Cardiol 2011;57: 160–6.
10. Berenfeld O, Mandapati R, Dixit S, et al. Spatially distributed dominant excitation frequencies reveal hidden organization in atrial fibrillation in the Langendorff-perfused sheep heart. J Cardiovasc Electrophysiol 2000;11:869–79.
11. Berenfeld O, Zaitsev AV, Mironov SF, et al. Frequency-dependent breakdown of wave propagation into fibrillatory conduction across the pectinate muscle network in the isolated sheep right atrium. Circ Res 2002;90:1173–80.

12. Kalifa J, Tanaka K, Zaitsev AV, et al. Mechanisms of wave fractionation at boundaries of high-frequency excitation in the posterior left atrium of the isolated sheep heart during atrial fibrillation. Circulation 2006;113:626–33.

13. Mandapati R, Skanes A, Chen J, et al. Stable microreentrant sources as a mechanism of atrial fibrillation in the isolated sheep heart. Circulation 2000;101:194–9.

14. Mansour M, Mandapati R, Berenfeld O, et al. Left-to-right gradient of atrial frequencies during acute atrial fibrillation in the isolated sheep heart. Circulation 2001;103:2631–6.

15. Skanes AC, Mandapati R, Berenfeld O, et al. Spatiotemporal periodicity during atrial fibrillation in the isolated sheep heart. Circulation 1998;98:1236–48.

16. Atienza F, Martins RP, Jalife J. Translational research in atrial fibrillation: a quest for mechanistically based diagnosis and therapy. Circ Arrhythm Electrophysiol 2012;5:1207–15.

17. Atienza F, Almendral J, Jalife J, et al. Real-time dominant frequency mapping and ablation of dominant frequency sites in atrial fibrillation with left-to-right frequency gradients predicts long-term maintenance of sinus rhythm. Heart Rhythm 2009;6:33–40.

18. Atienza F, Almendral J, Moreno J, et al. Activation of inward rectifier potassium channels accelerates atrial fibrillation in humans: evidence for a reentrant mechanism. Circulation 2006;114:2434–42.

19. Sanders P, Berenfeld O, Hocini M, et al. Spectral analysis identifies sites of high-frequency activity maintaining atrial fibrillation in humans. Circulation 2005;112:789–97.

20. Atienza F, Calvo D, Almendral J, et al. Mechanisms of fractionated electrograms formation in the posterior left atrium during paroxysmal atrial fibrillation in humans. J Am Coll Cardiol 2011;57:1081–92.

21. Jais P, Haissaguerre M, Shah DC, et al. A focal source of atrial fibrillation treated by discrete radiofrequency ablation. Circulation 1997;95:572–6.

22. Narayan SM, Krummen DE, Clopton P, et al. Direct or coincidental elimination of stable rotors or focal sources may explain successful atrial fibrillation ablation: on-treatment analysis of the confirm trial (conventional ablation for AF with or without focal impulse and rotor modulation). J Am Coll Cardiol 2013;62:138–47.

23. Narayan SM, Krummen DE, Shivkumar K, et al. Treatment of atrial fibrillation by the ablation of localized sources: CONFIRM (conventional ablation for atrial fibrillation with or without focal impulse and rotor modulation) trial. J Am Coll Cardiol 2012;60: 628–36.

24. Miller JM, Kowal RC, Swarup V, et al. Initial independent outcomes from focal impulse and rotor modulation ablation for atrial fibrillation: multicenter firm registry. J Cardiovasc Electrophysiol 2014;25: 921–9.

25. Dixit S, Gerstenfeld EP, Ratcliffe SJ, et al. Single procedure efficacy of isolating all versus arrhythmogenic pulmonary veins on long-term control of atrial fibrillation: a prospective randomized study. Heart Rhythm 2008;5:174–81.

26. Atienza F, Almendral J, Ormaetxe JM, et al. RADAR-AF Investigators. Multicenter comparison of radiofrequency catheter ablation of drivers versus circumferential pulmonary vein isolation in patients with atrial fibrillation. A noninferiority randomized clinical trial. J Am Coll Cardiol 2014, in press.

27. Gerstenfeld EP, SippensGroenewegen A, Lux RL, et al. Derivation of an optimal lead set for measuring ectopic atrial activation from the pulmonary veins by using body surface mapping. J Electrocardiol 2000; 33(Suppl):179–85.

28. Berenfeld O. Toward discerning the mechanisms of atrial fibrillation from surface electrocardiogram and spectral analysis. J Electrocardiol 2010;43: 509–14.

29. Guillem MS, Climent AM, Millet J, et al. Noninvasive localization of maximal frequency sites of atrial fibrillation by body surface potential mapping. Circ Arrhythm Electrophysiol 2013;6:294–301.

30. Rodrigo M, Guillem MS, Climent AM, et al. Body surface localization of left and right atrial high-frequency rotors in atrial fibrillation patients: a clinical-computational study. Heart Rhythm 2014; 11(9):1584–91.

31. Guillem MS, Climent AM, Castells F, et al. Noninvasive mapping of human atrial fibrillation. J Cardiovasc Electrophysiol 2009;20:507–13.

32. Berenfeld O. Quantifying activation frequency in atrial fibrillation to establish underlying mechanisms and ablation guidance. Heart Rhythm 2007;4:1225–34.

Comparative Analysis of Diagnostic 12-Lead Electrocardiography and 3-Dimensional Noninvasive Mapping

Kevin Ming Wei Leong, MBBS, MRCP, Phang Boon Lim, MA, MBBChir, MRCP, PhD, Prapa Kanagaratnam, MA, MBBChir, MRCP, PhD*

KEYWORDS

- Noninvasive mapping • 12-Lead electrocardiography • Body surface mapping
- Ventricular outflow tract tachycardia • Premature ventricular complex

KEY POINTS

- Noninvasive electrocardiographic mapping has accuracy superior to that of validated 12-lead electrogram algorithms in the localization of ventricular outflow tract arrhythmias.
- Noninvasive electrocardiographic mapping optimizes conventional pace and activation mapping techniques used to localize ectopy.
- The ability of noninvasive electrocardiographic mapping to rapidly and accurately localize ectopy origin from a single ectopic activation makes it particularly useful in patients with infrequent premature ventricular ectopy.

INTRODUCTION

Since the first human electrocardiogram (ECG) recorded by Waller in 1887, the 12-lead ECG has remained the standard tool to obtain electrophysiologic (EP) information from the heart noninvasively. Consequently, numerous ECG algorithms have been developed to assist electrophysiologists in localizing various atrial and ventricular arrhythmias, and accessory pathways (APs) to guide catheter ablation.[1–7]

Increasing the number of surface electrodes would be expected to increase the accuracy of determining the cardiac activation patterns, but requires appropriate methods to analyze the additional data. The validation of mathematical algorithms to reconstruct epicardial electrograms from body surface potentials led to the development and clinical demonstration of the noninvasive electrocardiographic mapping (ECM) system,[8] providing physicians with the ability to address the question of whether more surface-electrode information can lead to more accurate localization of tachycardias.

VENTRICULAR ARRHYTHMIAS OF THE OUTFLOW TRACT

Ventricular tachycardia (VT) or frequent premature ventricular complexes (PVCs) arising from the outflow tracts accounts for 10% of all VT,[9] and represent a particularly interesting group of patients in whom to study the value of ECM, as infrequent ectopy or difficulty inducing tachycardia

The authors have nothing to disclose.
Department of Cardiology, International Centre for Circulatory Health, St Mary's Hospital, Praed Street, Paddington, London W2 1NY, UK
* Corresponding author.
E-mail address: p.kanagaratnam@imperial.ac.uk

cardiacEP.theclinics.com

during the procedures is often the cause of limited success. Pace mapping using the surface ECG is central to the ablation procedure, and it is known that similar 12-lead ECG pace maps can be seen over a distance of 2 cm.

Most outflow tract VT (OTVT)/PVC has been demonstrated to arise from the anterior and superior septal aspect of the right ventricular outflow tract (RVOT), just inferior to the pulmonic valve.[10] It arises from the left ventricular outflow tract (LVOT) in approximately 10% to 15% of cases, where it can also be mapped to the region of the aortic cusps.[11] Much less commonly, it can also be localized to the right ventricular (RV) infundibulum, RV free wall, and posterior aspect of the interventricular septum.[2]

Catheter ablation within these complex anatomic structures can be effective in eliminating symptoms and reversing PVC-induced cardiomyopathy, but there remain significant limitations to current mapping techniques, including poor spatial resolution of pace mapping, inaccurate localization of VT origin based on ECG algorithms, and the lack of spontaneous ectopy rendering activation mapping ineffective.[12]

As OTVTs and PVCs usually arise from a single anatomic focus in a structurally normal heart, they are particularly amenable to localization with the 12-lead ECG. Accordingly ECG criteria have been extensively published, describing characteristics of ectopic foci originating from the RVOT and LVOT, in addition to the aortomitral continuity, anterior interventricular vein, and the aortic sinus cusps.[2,4,5,7,13]

A major limitation of algorithms designed to sublocalize the focus within the outflow tract is the derivation of these algorithms from pace mapping,[4,5,13] which has poor spatial resolution in the RVOT owing to its complex anatomy.[7,14] To improve the predictive accuracy in sublocalization, an ECG algorithm validated by noncontact electroanatomic mapping was developed by Zhang and colleagues.[7] The investigators reported a predictive accuracy of 88%,[7] although this was reported to be lower by another group.[12]

As algorithms become more specific at sublocalization, there are an increasing number of steps and measurements required to reach a diagnosis, thus increasing the chances of error and variability in results. Jamil-Copley and colleagues[12] observed that the reduction in the reliability of each algorithm was proportional to the number of steps needed to reach a diagnosis. For the algorithm used in their study, which involved 3 steps, there was 86% overall agreement between the 3 independent assessors, in contrast to a 43% overall agreement between assessors when an algorithm involving 5 steps was used.

Several of these algorithms require measurement of various ECG parameters, and consequential inconsistencies in measurement can arise when performed on a 12-lead ECG in the absence of electronic calipers. In addition, there is potential for error from a wandering baseline, lead noise, and absence of a suitable sinus rhythm beat preceding the PVC QRS, all of which are encountered in day-to-day clinical practice. Further inaccuracies in ECG algorithms are introduced by individual variability in the spatial relationship between the heart, thoracic wall, and overall body habitus among patients. Variable precordial lead placements can also yield confusing patterns.

The use of the ECM involves the patient wearing a vest of 252 electrodes and undergoing a low-resolution computed tomography (CT) scan. The reconstructed thorax with electrode localization is used as the model on which clinical VT/PVC morphologies are captured by the ECM system and processed to display potential and activation maps. The use of the patient's own cardiac anatomy from segmented CT geometry in the ECM system addresses the limitations set by individual variability and variable lead placement. This approach also makes the system highly accurate at localization, even in the presence of underlying structural cardiac abnormalities.

Localization of ectopy is based on the site of earliest epicardial breakthrough and subsequent activation sequence (**Fig. 1**). As the system in unable to track the catheter location in real time, a voltage map of the pacing spike can localize the pacing stimulus as a surrogate marker for catheter location (see **Fig. 1**), and can be used to guide the catheter toward the earliest site breakthrough. The ablation site is identified if:

1. The resultant potential and activation maps corresponds with those during the clinical VT/PVC
2. The catheter location on the voltage map corresponds anatomically with the earliest site of electrical activation

Jamil-Copley and colleagues[12] compared the accuracy of the noninvasive ECM system with that of validated ECG algorithms in localizing OTVT origin in patients undergoing ablation preprocedurally. The algorithms by Betensky and colleagues,[2] Zhang and colleagues,[7] and Ito and colleagues[4] were applied retrospectively to the ECGs showing the clinical VT/PVC, which were performed by 3 electrophysiologists who were blinded to the ECM data and ablation outcomes. ECM correctly identified the PVC origin

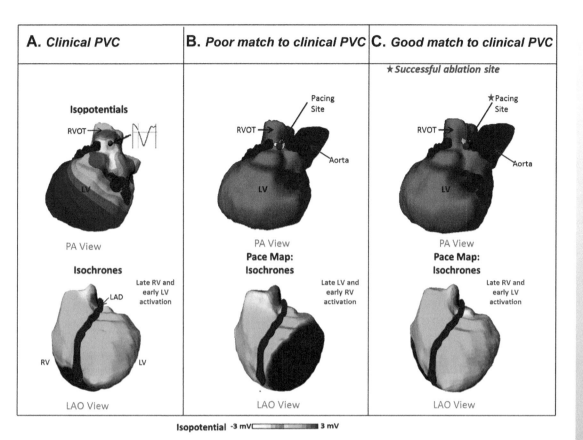

A. *Clinical PVC* | **B.** *Poor match to clinical PVC* | **C.** *Good match to clinical PVC*

★ *Successful ablation site*

Fig. 1. Electrocardiographic mapping (ECM) pacing spike voltage maps (*top*) and activation maps (*bottom*). (*A*) Clinical premature ventricular complex (PVC). (*B*) Pacing spike voltage and activation maps different from the clinical PVC. (*C*) Different pacing site location (*red dot*) with an activation map that looks similar to that of the clinical PVC. LAD, left anterior descending artery; LAO, left anterior oblique; LV, left ventricle; LVOT, left ventricular outflow tract; PA, posteroanterior; RV, right ventricle; RVOT, right ventricular outflow tract. (*From* Jamil-Copley S, Bokan R, Kojodjojo P, et al. Noninvasive electrocardiographic mapping to guide ablation of outflow tract ventricular arrhythmias. Heart Rhythm 2014;11;589; with permission.)

in 23 of the 24 cases. In 21 of these cases, identification was already made before commencement of the EP study from spontaneous PVC/VT preprocedurally. The remaining 3 were obtained periprocedurally.

There was accurate localization of the site of origin by the ECM system, as the first ablation lesion resulted in acute procedural success in all 23 patients (18 RV and 6 left ventricular sites: 3 posteroseptal RVOT, 8 anteroseptal RVOT, 4 midseptal RVOT, 2 posterolateral RVOT, 4 left coronary cusp, 1 noncoronary cusp/right coronary cusp junction, and 2 aortomitral continuity sites). Local bipolar electrogram at these sites during clinical ectopy also preceded VT/PVC QRS onset by 29 ± 9 milliseconds. In 22 of the 24 cases, a 12/12 pace match was achieved. The best pace maps at the remaining 2 sites were 11/12 and 10/12.

All patients had experienced significant improvement in symptoms in the immediate postoperative period. Twenty-one of the 24 patients remained symptom free or achieved reduction in symptom burden over a mean follow-up of 11 ± 4 months.

Comparison of Electrocardiogram Algorithms with Electrocardiographic Mapping in Localizing the Origin of Ventricular Tachycardia/Premature Ventricular Complex

Accurately predicting whether the arrhythmia is left-sided or right-sided is of importance, as it guides informed consent with regard to procedural time and risk. ECM accurately predicted the correct ventricular chamber in 96% of the cases, and successfully sublocalized the regions in all of them (100%).

The algorithm by Betensky and colleagues[2] uses a V2 transition ratio to predict a left versus right outflow tract origin (with a cutoff of $\geq$0.6 for left), and was reported to have a 91% accuracy. In study by Jamil-Copley and colleagues,[12] the predictive accuracy of an LVOT origin was much lower, varying between 67% and 71% between the 3 assessors, with an acceptable interrater agreement κ value of 0.72.

The algorithms by Zhang and colleagues[7] and Ito and colleagues[4] were also used in the study. These algorithms have not only the ability to differentiate LVOT from RVOT but can also sublocalize within the RVOT, with published sensitivity, specificity, and positive predictive values ranging from 79% to 95%.[4,7] When applied to the study's cohort of patients, the correct location (RV free wall vs RV septum vs left ventricle) was identified in only 46% to 63% of the cases, with poor interobserver agreement κ values of 0.15 and 0.54 for the algorithms, respectively.[12]

OTHER CHALLENGES IN THE MAPPING OF OUTFLOW TRACT VENTRICULAR TACHYCARDIA/PREMATURE VENTRICULAR COMPLEX AND THE ELECTROCARDIOGRAPHIC MAPPING SYSTEM
Pace Mapping

Localization of the OTVT/PVC origin can be achieved by pace mapping the region of interest identified by the 12-lead ECG, with the aim achieving an exact 12-lead match with spontaneous OTVT/PVC.[15] However, this mapping technique can be imprecise, as it has been shown that exact matches can still be achieved from pacing sites more than 2 cm away from the origin of the PVC, suggesting reduced specificity and spatial resolution.[16]

Pace mapping may also have difficulty locating foci deep within the myocardial wall. The activation wave front from such an origin reaches the endocardial surface by conduction through preferential fibers. Hence, when pacing is performed at the earliest site endocardial activation, capture of the myocardium surrounding the catheter tip may result in a QRS complex that reflects local capture and that differs from the native QRS complex of the PVC/VT.[14]

Despite its limitations, pace mapping is a practical method of localizing the site of origin in situations where VT/PVCs are infrequent and not reproducibly inducible. Three-dimensional (3D) electroanatomic maps from the ECM system of a single ectopic beat can guide the catheter to the region of interest quickly by pace-spike mapping (see **Fig. 1**), potentially reducing the procedural time it requires an operator to reach the site where the best pace-mapping match can be achieved.

Activation Mapping

Activation mapping using unipolar and bipolar ECGs can also be used to corroborate the pace map findings in patients with frequent OTVT/PVC. Successful catheter ablation has been shown to be more positively correlated with sites of earliest activation when compared with sites with good pace maps (quantified as having 11 or 12 out of 12 matching leads).[14]

However, the mean area of myocardium activated within the first 10 milliseconds during RVOT VT can range from 1.3 to 6.4 cm^2. Bearing in mind that the lesion created by a catheter tip is less than 1.2 cm^2, ablation at any single site within the 10M isochrone would not be expected to be effective. Along with an interobserver variability of up to 5 milliseconds or more in the manual assignment of activation time, this compounds the limitation of activation mapping. Furthermore, sequential activation mapping is depends heavily on sufficient spontaneous clinical ectopy.

A global 3D display of activation times allows comparison of data from nearby sites, overcoming the imprecision of assigned activation times at single points, and permits rapid identification of a putative site of origin in the center of the earliest activation area. The Ensite array is an invasive noncontact mapping technique that provides 3D electroanatomic maps and allows for mapping of single beats of ectopy. However, it requires systemic heparinization, even in the right ventricle, increasing the risk of bleeding complications. Furthermore, only a single chamber can be mapped at a time.

Such limitations are overcome by the noninvasive ECM system that can simultaneously provide electroanatomic maps over both ventricles. Patients can also remain ambulant for several hours before the EP study to allow spontaneous arrhythmia to be recorded without prolonging invasive procedural time. Individuals are also able to undertake maneuvers outside the EP laboratory to induce ectopy, which include aerobic exercises on the treadmill. Potential shifts in geometry can be avoided by creating the ECM maps after peak exercise with the patient in the recumbent position.[12]

ATRIAL TACHYCARDIAS

Atrial tachycardia (AT) accounts for 5% to 15% of all supraventricular tachycardias, and can occur in the presence or absence of structural heart disease. The foci of origin are distributed throughout the atria and are most commonly found at the pulmonary veins, crista terminalis, coronary sinus, and atrial septum.[6] Prolonged episodes of AT (usually months or years) can result in negative remodeling of the atria and ventricles, causing myopathy and symptoms of congestive heart failure. These arrhythmias are amenable to ablation, which if performed early can prevent such irreversible changes.

ECG algorithms for localizing AT are based on the interpretation of P-wave morphology, and have a reported sensitivity and specificity ranging from 88% to 93% and 79% to 83%, respectively.[6,17,18] Predictive accuracy deteriorates when applied to patients with enlarged atria as the anatomic relationship between the atria changes, in patients with previous ablations and in scenarios where AT arises from uncommon sites (eg, left atrial septum and vena cava).

The use of the ECM system in mapping AT has been validated during invasive catheter mapping and ablation.[19] In this multicenter study involving 48 patients, ECM successfully localized and identified the mechanism of AT in 92% of the participants. The study cohort included simple and complex ATs, and patients with previous atrial surgery and ablation. The study showed that ECM has an 85% diagnostic accuracy for macroreentrant circuits (eg, perimitral, cavotricuspid isthmus-dependent, roof-dependent, around surgical scar), and a 100% localization accuracy for focal ATs.[19]

Superior usefulness of the ECM system over the ECG in mapping ATs is demonstrated in various case reports.[20,21] Previous cardiothoracic surgery and atrial scarring are some of the scenarios in which interpretation of the P-wave morphology becomes unreliable and where the ECM possesses greater clinical utility. Deterioration of P-wave morphology was noted in a patient with AT who had previously undergone pulmonary vein isolation and was not amenable to mapping with the ECG.[20] In this case report the ECM system located the focus to the superior left atrium between the right superior pulmonary vein and the atrial septum, resulting in a successful ablation.

Cakulev and colleagues[21] provided 2 examples after cardiothoracic surgery whereby the P-wave morphologies on ECG could not suggest a particular site of origin or mechanism of the tachyarrhythmia. In the first case, the ECM successfully identified a focus in the left atrium, and was subsequently confirmed as a left-sided focal AT on EP study. In the second case, ECM elucidated a right-sided cavo-tricuspid-isthmus–dependent reentrant circuit that was not readily clear on the ECG.[21]

ACCESSORY PATHWAYS

Since Rosenbaum first attempted to localize APs to either the left or right atrioventricular ring using the 12-lead ECG, several algorithms have been developed to more precisely locate APs based on QRS and delta-wave morphology.[3]

One such algorithm by Arruda and colleagues[1] has sensitivity of 90% and specificity of 99%, but is reportedly much lower in the pediatric population.[3] The presence of congenital/structural heart disease or multiple pathways have also been shown to reduce the predictive accuracy of the algorithm.[3]

Ghosh and colleagues[22] investigated the phenomenon of cardiac memory in 14 pediatric patients with Wolff-Parkinson-White syndrome undergoing catheter ablation. The ECM system and the algorithm by Arruda and colleagues[1] were both used to localize the APs, although it is unclear from the article if operators of the algorithm were blinded to ECM data and ablation outcome. **Table 1** provides a summary of their findings.

All 14 patients had their APs successfully ablated, with the ECM system correctly identifying the location in all of them. The algorithm correctly predicted the location in 13 of 14 patients. In 3 (21%) cases (subjects 3, 4, and 6 in **Table 1**), the investigators report an improvement in pathway localization with the ECM system over the algorithm. The ECM identified multiple pathways in one, an epicardial origin in another, and correctly predicted a right-sided pathway, which was predicted to be on either side based on the algorithm.

Cakulev and colleagues[21] also similarly reported on the ability of the ECM to correctly predict a left-sided or right-sided AP in 4 patients, in whom the ECG was indeterminate in predicting the location of the AP.

LIMITATIONS OF ELECTROCARDIOGRAPHIC MAPPING

A potential weakness of the ECM system is that it derives its information from reconstructed ECGs on the epicardial surface of the heart. The endocardial sequence of activation will not always be identical to the epicardial activation sequence, although a recent report has shown close correlation between invasive endocardial mapping and noninvasive ECM epicardial imaging.[23]

With arrhythmias arising from the septum, it can be difficult to tell whether earliest activation is on the right of left just by looking at the reconstructed

Table 1
Accessory pathway (AP) location by electrocardiographic mapping (ECM) system, 12-lead electrocardiogram (ECG), and site of successful ablation

Patient	Age (y)	ECM Prediction of AP Location	ECG Prediction of AP Location	Site of Successful Ablation
1	12	7:00, MA, endo	LAL, LL	7:00, MA, endo
2	16	4:00, MA, endo	LAL, LL	4:00, MA, endo
3	5	2 APs: 3:00 and 5:00, MA, endo	LAL, LL	2 sites: 3:00 and 5:00, MA, endo
4	13	5:00, TA, endo	PSTA, PSMA	5:00, TA, endo
5	12	4:00, TA or 8:00 MA, endo	PSTA, PSMA	3:00, TA, endo
6	13	7:00, MA, epi	PSTA	7:00, MA, epi
7	8	7:00, MA, endo	LPL, LP	7:00, MA, endo
8	13	3:00, TA or 9:00 MA, endo	PSTA, PSMA	3:00, TA, endo
9	10	7:00, MA, endo	LPL, LP	7:00, MA, endo
10	15	6:00, MA, endo	LPL, LP	6:00, MA, endo
11	13	6:00, TA, endo	RP, RPL	6:00, TA, endo
12	12	3:00, MA, endo	LL, LAL	3:00, MA, endo
13	12	5:00, MA, endo	LAL, LL	5:00, MA, endo
14	10	5:00, TA, epi	MCV or venous anomaly	5:00, TA, epi

7:00, 4:00, 3:00, 5:00, 6:00, 8:00, and 9:00 refer, under left anterior oblique view, to 7 o'clock position, 4 o'clock position, 3 o'clock position, and so forth.

Abbreviations: endo, endocardial; epi, epicardial; LAL, left anterolateral; LL, left lateral; LP, left posterior; LPL, left posterolateral; MA, mitral annulus; MCV, middle cardiac vein; PSMA, posteroseptal mitral annulus; PSTA, posteroseptal tricuspid annulus; RP, right posterior; RPL, right posterolateral; TA, tricuspid annulus.

Adapted from Ghosh S, Rhee EK, Avari JN, et al. Cardiac memory in patients with Wolff-Parkinson-White syndrome: noninvasive imaging of activation and repolarisation before and after catheter ablation. Circulation 2008;118:907–15.

ECGs. Studies reporting the interobserver variability in interpretation have yet to be published. The ECM method used to localize ectopy origin (**Fig. 2**) provides a useful way to differentiate, although like any other mapping system it does not provide complete predictive accuracy. In one case in the study by Jamil-Copley and colleagues,[12] the ECM method predicted a septal

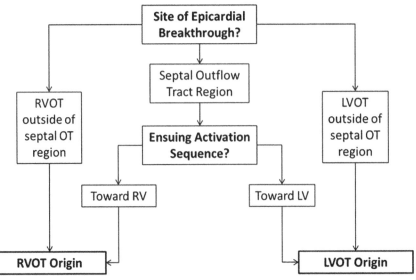

Fig. 2. Localization of ectopy using the ECM system. (*Adapted from* Jamil-Copley S, Bokan R, Kojodjojo P, et al. Noninvasive electrocardiographic mapping to guide ablation of outflow tract ventricular arrhythmias. Heart Rhythm 2014;11:587–94.)

RVOT origin but was later found to originate between the right and noncoronary cusp of the LVOT.

Of importance is that ECM requires a CT scan of the thorax with a mean radiation exposure of 148 mGy/cm. This exposure needs to be weighed against the benefits of accurate localization of the arrhythmia or pathway, and the potential reduction in procedural and fluoroscopic time. Future technological advances may allow cardiac MRI to replace the CT scan for anatomic correlation.

SUMMARY

Noninvasive ECM is superior to validated 12-lead ECG algorithms in identifying OTVT origin in guiding catheter ablation. The ECM system potentially has a higher clinical value in the localization of APs and atrial arrhythmias, and overcomes many of the limitations associated with conventional mapping techniques.

REFERENCES

1. Arruda MS, McClelland JH, Wang X, et al. Development and validation of an ECG algorithm for identifying accessory pathway ablation site in Wolff-Parkinson-White Syndrome. J Cardiovasc Electrophysiol 1998; 9:2–12.
2. Betensky BP, Park RE, Marchlinski FE, et al. The V2 transition ratio: a new electrocardiographic criterion for distinguishing left from right ventricular outflow tract tachycardia origin. J Am Coll Cardiol 2011;57: 2255–62.
3. Bar-Cohen Y, Khairy P, Morwood J, et al. Inaccuracy of Wolff-Parkinson-White accessory pathway localization algorithms in children and patients with congenital heart defects. J Cardiovasc Electrophysiol 2006;17:712–6.
4. Ito S, Tada H, Naito S, et al. Development and validation of an ECG algorithm for identifying the optimal ablation site for idiopathic ventricular outflow tract tachycardia. J Cardiovasc Electrophysiol 2003; 14:1280–6.
5. Joshi S, Wilber D. Ablation of idiopathic right ventricular outflow tract tachycardia-current perspectives. J Cardiovasc Electrophysiol 2005;16:S52–8.
6. Qian ZY, Hou XF, Xu DJ, et al. An algorithm to predict the site of origin of focal atrial tachycardia. Pacing Clin Electrophysiol 2011;34:414–21.
7. Zhang F, Chen M, Yang B, et al. Electrocardiographic algorithm to identify the optimal target ablation site for idiopathic right ventricular outflow tract ventricular premature contraction. Europace 2009; 11:1214–20.
8. Ramanathan C, Jia P, Ghanem R, et al. Activation and repolarization of the normal heart under complete physiological conditions. Proc Natl Acad Sci U S A 2006;103:6309–14.
9. Aliot E, Stevenson G, Amendral-Garrote J, et al. EHRA/HRS Expert consensus on catheter ablation of ventricular arrhythmias. Europace 2009;11: 771–817.
10. Movsowitz C, Schwartzman D, Callans DJ, et al. Idiopathic right ventricular outflow tract tachycardia: narrowing the anatomic location for successful ablation. Am Heart J 1996;131:930–6.
11. Callans DJ, Menz V, Schwartzman D, et al. Repetitive monomorphic tachycardia from the left ventricular outflow tract: electrocardiographic patterns consistent with a left ventricular site of origin. J Am Coll Cardiol 1997;29:1023–7.
12. Jamil-Copley S, Bokan R, Kojodjojo P, et al. Noninvasive electrocardiographic mapping to guide ablation of outflow tract ventricular arrhythmias. Heart Rhythm 2014;11:587–94.
13. Dixit S, Gerstenfeld EP, Callans DJ, et al. Electrocardiographic patterns of superior right ventricular outflow tract tachycardias distinguishing septal and free-wall origin. J Cardiovasc Electrophysiol 2003;14:1–7.
14. Bogun F, Taj M, Ting M, et al. Spatial resolution of pace-mapping of idiopathic ventricular tachycardia/ectopy originating in the right ventricular outflow tract. Heart Rhythm 2008;5:39–44.
15. Bala R, Marchlinski F. Electrocardiographic recognition and ablation of outflow tract ventricular tachycardia. Heart Rhythm 2007;4:366–70.
16. Azegami K, Wilber DJ, Aarruda M, et al. Spatial resolution of pace-mapping and activation mapping inpatients with idiopathic right ventricular outflow tract tachycardia. J Am Coll Cardiol 2005; 39:1808–12.
17. Tang CW, Scheinman MM, Van Hare GF, et al. Use of P wave configuration during atrial tachycardia to predict site of origin. J Am Coll Cardiol 1995;26: 1315–24.
18. Kistler PM, Roberts-Thomson KC, Haqqani HM, et al. P-wave morphology in focal atrial tachycardia: development of an algorithm to predict the anatomic site of origin. J Am Coll Cardiol 2006;48:1010–7.
19. Shah AJ, Hocini M, Xhaet O, et al. Validation of novel 3-dimensional electrocardiographic mapping of atrial tachycardias by invasive mapping and ablation. J Am Coll Cardiol 2013;62:889–97.
20. Wang Y, Cuculich PS, Woodward PK, et al. Focal atrial tachycardia after pulmonary vein isolation: noninvasive mapping with electrocardiographic imaging. Heart Rhythm 2007;4:1081–4.
21. Cakulev I, Sahadevan J, Arruda M, et al. Confirmation of novel noninvasive high-density electrocardiographic mapping with electrophysiology study: implications for therapy. Circ Arrhythm Electrophysiol 2013;6:68–75.

22. Ghosh S, Rhee EK, Avari JN, et al. Cardiac memory in patients with Wolff-Parkinson-White syndrome: noninvasive imaging of activation and repolarisation before and after catheter ablation. Circulation 2008;118:907–15.

23. Wang Y, Cuculich PS, Zhang J, et al. Noninvasive electroanatomical mapping of human ventricular arrhythmias with electrocardiographic imaging. Sci Transl Med 2011;3:98.

Noninvasive Diagnostic Mapping of Supraventricular Arrhythmias (Wolf-Parkinson-White Syndrome and Atrial Arrhythmias)

Ivan Cakulev, MD[a],*, Jayakumar Sahadevan, MD[b], Albert L. Waldo, MD[a]

KEYWORDS

- Noninvasive mapping • WPW • Atrial arrhythmias • Body surface mapping
- Cardiac electroanatomic mapping

KEY POINTS

- Twelve-lead electrocardiograms (ECGs) have limited value in predicting the origin and mechanism of focal or reentrant atrial arrhythmias, as well as precisely locating the ventricular insertion of accessory atrioventricular (AV) conduction pathways.
- Current clinical data suggest that it is possible to noninvasively determine with great accuracy the mechanism of the arrhythmia, the location of the focus or the accessory AV conduction, and the critical component of the reentrant circuit.
- On the basis of the noninvasive mapping data, the invasive procedure may be more focused, faster, easier, and safer.
- The current system can be especially helpful in patients who have failed previous ablation and in circumstances in which unusual and difficult anatomy is present or expected.
- The potential advantages of the system can help plan the invasive electrophysiological procedure, counsel the patient regarding the risk of the procedure but require an imaging study to be done before the invasive study.

INTRODUCTION

Although the 12-lead ECG is widely used and its efficacy recognized, the existence of only 6 leads covering a limited precordial area led several researchers to suggest several alternatives to more accurately record epicardial electrical activity.[1,2]

It is beyond the scope of this article to provide historical and detailed reviews of different systems designed in the last few decades to noninvasively

A.L. Waldo MD, PhD (Hon), is a consultant for CardioInsight Technologies, Inc., Cleveland, OH, USA. I. Cakulev, MD, and J. Sahadevan, MD, have nothing to disclose.
[a] Division of Cardiovascular Medicine, Department of Medicine, Harrington Heart & Vascular Institute, University Hospitals Case Medical Center, 11100 Euclid Avenue, MS LKS 5038, Cleveland, OH 44106, USA; [b] Department of Cardiology, Louis Stokes Cleveland Veterans Affairs Medical Center, 10701 East Boulevard, Cleveland, OH 44106, USA
* Corresponding author.
E-mail address: Ivan.Cakulev@case.edu

Card Electrophysiol Clin 7 (2015) 79–88
http://dx.doi.org/10.1016/j.ccep.2014.11.005

cardiacEP.theclinics.com

record epicardial electrical activation. In brief, the following systems are available:

1. Body surface potential mapping (BSPM): This is the first and one of the most widely studied alternatives to the 12-lead ECG in clinical and experimental electrocardiology. This system incorporates anywhere from 16 to 256 torso electrodes to record the electrocardiographic information as projected onto the body's surface. Unipolar potentials of single heartbeats are acquired simultaneously from all the torso electrodes. The amplitude of every electrogram is measured at a given time instant during the cardiac cycle and plotted on a chart representing the torso surface. At least 20 to 50 properly selected maps are sufficient to show the essential features of the time-varying surface field. Despite hundreds of studies that have demonstrated higher diagnostic and prognostic information than can be elicited from the 12-lead ECG, BSPM has not become a routinely used clinical method. One reason is that visual examination is complicated, relies on comparing each individual map to maps of normal patients, and memorization of different patterns and variability between normal subjects and patients becomes cumbersome. BSPM does not permit inferring the sequence of excitation and repolarization in the heart with a sufficient degree of certainty and detail because of the remote locations of the body surface electrodes relative to the heart and the torso volume conductor that acts as a filler to smooth the potentials.
2. Electrocardiographic imaging (ECGI) has been commercialized by CardioInsight Technologies Inc. (Cleveland, OH, USA) under the name of EC-VUE. In many reports, the term ECM (electrocardiographic mapping) is used to refer to this system. In order to overcome the limitations of BSPM, the system solves the so-called "electrocardiographic inverse problem" to estimate the equivalent cardiac sources from body surface potentials. In addition, the system uses a multielectrode electrocardiographic vest with a multichannel mapping system for ECG signal acquisition and an anatomic imaging modality, computed tomography (CT), to determine the heart-torso geometry. This makes it possible to image potentials, electrograms, and activation sequences (isochrones) on the epicardium in a unique fashion to generate noninvasive images of cardiac electrical activity.[3]
3. Noninvasive imaging of cardiac electrophysiology (NICE) uses 65 electrodes and a cardiac MRI to define the ventricular end-diastolic geometry and torso geometry.[4] Although endocardial and epicardial ventricular activation can be visualized noninvasively, the atrial activation cannot be analyzed using the NICE technique, and also, the model does not account for ventricular repolarization.
4. AMYCARD uses 83 electrodes and CT or MRI to image the torso anatomy.[5] It has been commercialized by AMYCARD LLC (Moscow, Russia). Because AMYCARD has only recently been installed in several Russian research centers, no data on the accuracy of this technique are yet available.

NONINVASIVE MAPPING IN SPECIFIC SUPRAVENTRICULAR SYNDROMES
Noninvasive Mapping of Atrial and Ventricular Insertion in Accessory Atrioventricular Connection

The location of the ventricular and atrial insertion of the accessory atrioventricular connection (AACV) has always been of paramount importance in treating patients with symptomatic Wolf-Parkinson-White (WPW) syndrome.

The first documented use of noninvasive mapping in human subjects with WPW syndrome dates back to 1975.[6] BSPM with 89 electrodes was used in 22 subjects to correlate the body surface isopotential maps with the patterns on the 12-lead ECG. Subsequently, other reports using BSPM stressed the correlation between the body surface minimum potential and the general location of the earliest site of ventricular preexcitation.[7,8] Other authors distinguished several patterns of body surface potentials that correlated with the location of the AACV as determined by multicatheter electrophysiologic study or surgical ablation of the AACV.[9] The few studies using BSPM to detect the location of the AACV had several issues: location of the AACV was not described in a standard fashion amongst the different studies; many of the studies used general locations (right/left anterior, posterior, lateral locations) without sufficient resolution; disagreement existed as to the timing—when exactly into the delta waves the analysis of the potential distribution should commence. Many groups analyzed only at 1 point, some scanned the whole QRS complex and ST-T interval; many of the study subjects did not have full ventricular preexcitation during the analysis, and only in some was atrial pacing or adenosine used during BSPM analysis. To avoid the instability of the QRS distributions during the delta wave, some groups recommended that an amplitude-based rather than a time-based criterion be used in determining which BSPMs should be analyzed. No standard equipment in relation to the number of electrodes or software for analysis was used.

In 1991, our laboratory reported the results of BSPM using 180 electrodes in 34 patients with WPW syndrome.[10] All 34 patients had an electrophysiologic study (EPS), and 18 had surgery, during which the ventricular insertion sites were accurately located using EPS/mapping. In order to standardize the location of the AACVs and improve the location accuracy, an anatomic grid (described by Guiraudon) with 17 ventricular insertion sites, each approximately 1.5 cm from each other, was used.[11] The ventricular insertion sites of AACVs determined by BSPM and by EPS at surgery were identical in all but 4 of the 18 patients; 3 of the 4 exceptions had more than one AACV, and the fourth had a broad ventricular insertion. Furthermore, it was concluded that standard electrocardiography using the Gallagher grid methodology[12] was not as accurate as QRS analysis of BSPM in predicting the ventricular insertion sites of AACVs. Importantly, BSPM appeared to be very accurate in predicting left versus right posteroseptal insertions of the AACVs.

The cumbersome, complex, and difficult-to-interpret results of BSPM, along with subsequent expansion and refinement of catheter-driven endocardial mapping techniques, and development of relatively accurate ECG criteria to localize AACVs resulted in abandonment of BSPM. The technique is no longer used to obtain clinical data in human subjects.

Although considerable experience was gained with catheter-based EPS, and relatively accurate depictions of the ventricular insertion site of AACVs were made possible by using 3-dimensional electroanatomic and activation maps, the approach was invasive and had well-recognized limitations. During this time, the efforts to improve the technology to noninvasively study epicardial cardiac activation continued. In 2006, Berger reported the results of NICE mapping in 7 patients with WPW syndrome undergoing catheter ablation.[13] The patients' cardiac anatomy was obtained by magnetic resonance imaging (MRI), and the NICE results were correlated with the successful ablation site identified by electroanatomic mapping (CARTO; Biosense Webster, Diamond Bar, CA, USA). All ventricular AACV insertion sites were identified with an accuracy of 18.7 ± 5.8 mm (at baseline) and 18.7 ± 6.4 mm (after adenosine administration). Although this was the first report to accurately and visually present the ventricular insertion site of an AACV by noninvasively combining the cardiac anatomy obtained by MRI and the electrical information obtained from the body surface, it was not followed by larger cohorts of patients and was not validated in other laboratories.

In 2008, Ghosh reported the use of ECGI in 14 pediatric patients with WPW syndrome that were imaged with ECGI a day before, at 45 minutes, 1 week, and 1 month after successful catheter ablation. ECGI determined that ventricular preexcitation sites were consistent with sites of successful ablation in all cases. The system was able to identify the presence of multiple pathways in 1 subject (2 separate and simultaneous activations) and the presence of an epicardial pathway. The latter is accomplished by analyzing the unipolar signals at the earliest (breakthrough) ventricular site of activation. When compared to the 12-lead ECG–based Arruda algorithm,[14] the system was better in 3 of 14 patients (21% improvement in accuracy). ECGI maps of retrograde atrial activation were also constructed in 5 subjects in whom a clear retrograde P wave was discerned after the QRS on the body-surface ECG during SVT. Examples of ECGI activation maps during SVT are shown in **Fig. 1** for a left-sided and a right-sided pathway. Ventricular repolarization can readily be studied with the system, and in this report, ventricular repolarization changes and spatial dispersion of repolarization changes as a result of the presence of the AACV persisted for 1 month after successful ablation.

Using the same system and technology, we reported our experience in 27 patients with various atrial and ventricular rhythm disorders.[15] Of 6 patients with WPW syndrome, 4 had ECGs suggestive of a septal ventricular insertion of the AACV per published 12-lead ECG–based algorithms.[14] In all of these patients, the ECG was indeterminate as far as whether the ventricular insertion was on the left or right side of the ventricular septum. In these patients, ECM accurately predicted whether the ventricular insertion of the AACV was in the left or the right ventricle, which was confirmed by the EPS/mapping. One of these 4 patients had an epicardial insertion of the pathway that was accurately identified by ECM. A representative example is shown in **Fig. 2**.

The Bordeaux group has used the same system in patients with WPW syndrome who had previously failed multiple ablations.[16] In this report, the system enabled the localization of AACVs of unusual location and their relationship with surrounding anatomic structures, as well as the scarring from prior ablation procedures. A representative example is shown in **Fig. 3**. The researchers concluded that "in the setting of WPW syndrome that is resistant to ablation, our results support the use of noninvasive testing to characterize accessory pathways that are frequently of unusual location."

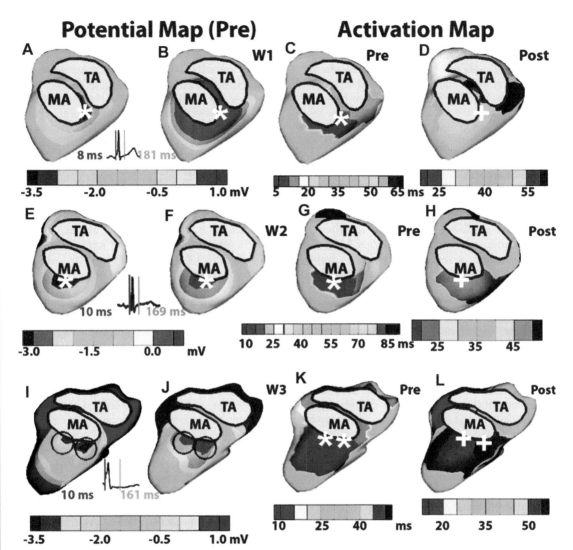

Fig. 1. ECGI-imaged epicardial voltage maps (left 2 panels, both before ablation) and activation maps (right 2 panels, before and after ablation, respectively) in subjects W1, W2, and W3 arranged in 3 rows, each row corresponding to 1 subject. The maps are presented in the left posterior view. (*A, E*) Epicardial potential minimum (*deep blue, asterisk*) associated with epicardial breakthrough early (8 and 10 ms) after onset of the delta wave. (*B, F*) Corresponding potential maximum (*red, asterisk*) during early repolarization. ECG lead V2 is shown for timing. The spatial pattern of epicardial potentials during early repolarization follows the pattern during early activation with reverse polarity, indicating the presence of an activation source at or below the site of epicardial breakthrough. In the third row, the preablation epicardial potential map in subject W3 shows 2 discrete potential minima (*I; blue, circles*) during early activation and 2 discrete potential maxima at the corresponding sites (*J; red, circles*) during early repolarization, indicating the presence of 2 activation sources (APs) in close proximity. The third column shows ECGI-imaged epicardial activation maps (isochrones) with the area of earliest activation in red (initiation site marked by *asterisk*). The fourth column shows the epicardial activation map 45 minutes after ablation; activation of the preablation preexcitation region now occurs late (*blue, +*). (*From* Ghosh S, Rhee EK, Avari JN, et al. Cardiac memory in patients with Wolff-Parkinson-White syndrome: noninvasive imaging of activation and repolarization before and after catheter ablation. Circulation 2008;118(9):907–15; with permission.)

Noninvasive Mapping of Atrial Tachycardia and Atrial Flutter

Atrial tachyarrhythmias represent the most common clinical heart rhythm disorder. Twelve-lead ECG is the standard-of-care technology to diagnose the origin of atrial tachyarrhythmias but has its limits in diagnosing the mechanisms and locations of the arrhythmia, especially in subjects

A

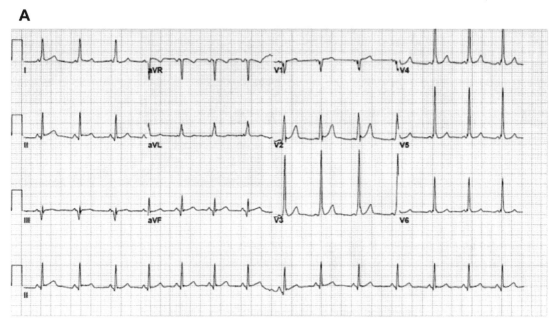

B

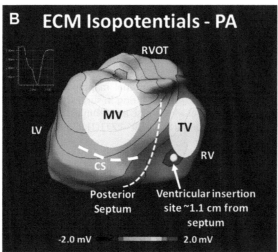

Fig. 2. (*A*) A 12-lead ECG of a 35-year-old man with ventricular preexcitation. Two features are worth mentioning. The first is that the transition in the precordial leads is between V1 and V2. The insertion could be either on the right side or the left side of the ventricular, although a larger R wave than S wave in lead I may suggest a right-sided pathway. The second feature is that the ECG is not fully preexcited, which again often adds to the ambiguity in determining the ventricular insertion site from the 12-lead ECG. (*B*) The ECM isopotential map shows that the site of earliest activation or the ventricular insertion site of the accessory pathway is approximately 1.1 cm off the ventricular septum on the right side. The recording of the electrogram from this earliest site of activation in the ventricles is also shown. This was also the site of successful ablation.

with previous ablation, and requires use of complex algorithms. Technological advances have resulted in the development of sophisticated 3-dimensional mapping systems that have helped in understanding and treating the arrhythmias, but we still rely on serial, beat-by-beat sequence-activation arrhythmia mapping, which can be time consuming and can be done only during the invasive procedure. Because of these limitations,

attempts to design a high-density noninvasive mapping system have remained an important goal in the last 4 decades.

The earliest attempts to map atrial arrhythmias were again done with BSPM. BSPM was used in several studies to obtain improved spatial resolution in discriminating focal atrial activity. These studies initially involved multisite pacing of the atria, creating atlases of maps corresponding to the

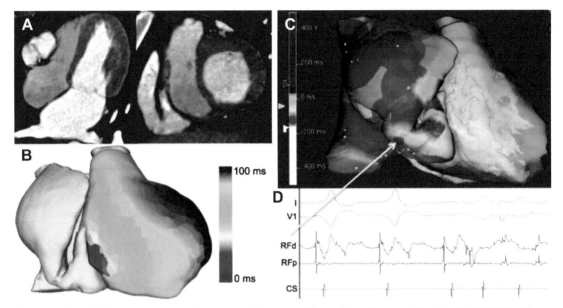

Fig. 3. Multimodality assessment and catheter ablation guidance in a 14-year-old girl with Wolff-Parkinson-White syndrome that was resistant to prior ablation. The patient experienced 2 sudden cardiac arrests related to VF episodes. The surface 12-lead ECG showed right-sided ventricular preexcitation resistant to 3 ablation procedures, including one with an epicardial approach. (*A*) Contrast-enhanced ECG-gated cardiac multidetector CT showed a right-atrium diverticulum emerging from the inferior insertion of the right appendage and extending toward right ventricular free wall. (*B*) These anatomic data were combined with the ventricular activation data acquired by using BSM and demonstrated that the diverticulum was hosting the accessory pathway. (*C*) The patient-specific model was integrated into a 3-dimensional mapping system to guide the ablation. Ablation was performed at the diverticulum ostium (*arrow*), resulting in successful termination of (*D*) ventricular preexcitation. (*From* Cochet H, Dubois R, Sacher F, et al. Cardiac arrhythmias: multimodal assessment integrating body surface ECG mapping into cardiac imaging. Radiology 2014;271(1):239–47; with permission.)

individual paced atrial sites. These maps were then compared with the maps of patients undergoing invasive studies for atrial arrhythmias.[17,18] Although clinical accuracy was determined for localizing right atrial foci, it was not possible to report whether BSPM could successfully differentiate between left- and right-sided ectopic atrial arrhythmias. The same group also studied BSPM in typical and reverse typical (counterclockwise and clockwise) atrial flutter.[19] BSPM with 62 surface electrodes was used in 20 patients with isthmus-dependent atrial flutter. BSPM allowed for direct correlations of the instantaneous surface map pattern during a given period in the atrial flutter wave cycle, with activation of distinct components in the right atrial macro-reentrant circuit. Reported BSPM efforts to define atrial arrhythmias are few, and results do not allow for concluding that the mechanism and the precise location of the arrhythmia can be elicited with BSPM. Consequently, this system is currently not clinically used.

Using ECGI, case reports showed feasibility of mapping typical isthmus-dependent and atypical atrial flutter.[3,20] Because the system used

high-density recording, needed only 1 beat for analysis, provided activation times superimposed on the cardiac anatomic shell derived from CT imaging, and showed promise in eliciting the mechanism and defining the location of the arrhythmia, our group used it in patients with various atrial and ventricular arrhythmias.[15] In this report, in all 10 patients with an atrial tachyarrhythmia, ECM was able to identify whether the arrhythmia was coming from the left or right atrium and whether the arrhythmia was focal or reentrant. Five patients in this group had an atrial tachycardia (AT) involving the left atrium. Representative examples are shown in **Figs. 4** and **5**.

The most robust and clinically relevant use of noninvasive mapping in atrial arrhythmias was reported in 2013.[21] Fifty-two patients with clinical AT, including patients who previously underwent extensive ablation for atrial fibrillation (AF), and patients from 3 centers (in France and the United States) who had an atriotomy were analyzed using ECM. Structural heart disease was present in 35%, and 52% had a previous AF ablation. The accuracy of ECM in diagnosing the arrhythmia mechanism and locating the arrhythmia during

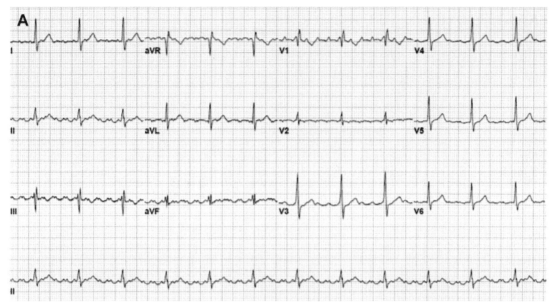

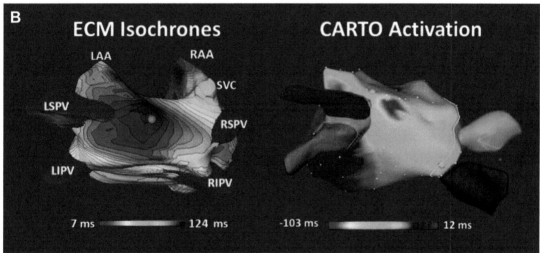

Fig. 4. (A) ECG of a 72-year-old man after a single lung transplant for idiopathic pulmonary fibrosis. He had inces-
sant atrial tachycardia that was not controlled with multiple antiarrhythmic medications. The ECG shows an atrial
tachycardia with a P wave morphology that does not suggested any particular site of origin. Note the lack of an
isoelectric interval between the P waves, which may suggest a reentrant mechanism of the arrhythmia. (B) On the
left side of the figure, the ECM map demonstrated focal activation of the left atrium, with the earliest site of
activation on the left atrial roof. This area was close to the atrial incision that was made during the left lung
transplant. The right side of the figure shows the CARTO map with the successful site of ablation that terminated
the tachycardia and rendered it noninducible. As can be appreciated, the ECM site of earliest activation matches
the site of successful ablation. The activation pattern demonstrates focal activation of the left atrium. LAA, left
atrial appendage; LIPV, left inferior pulmonary vein; LSPV, left superior pulmonary vein; RIPV, right inferior pulmonary vein; RSPV, right superior pulmonary vein; SVC, superior vena cava.

AT was determined by comparison with invasive
mapping and confirmed by successful ablation
in all patients. Out of 48 clinical ATs, 27 were
diagnosed in the electrophysiology (EP) laboratory as macro-reentrant and 21 as focal arrhythmias. ECM identified the mechanism of AT as
macro-reentry versus focal activation in 44 of
48 (92%) patients. Among 27 patients with
macro-reentrant AT diagnosed invasively, there
were 18 cavotricuspid isthmus-dependent, 5
perimitral, and 3 roof-dependent ATs. In addition, 1 AT was reentry around the right atrial

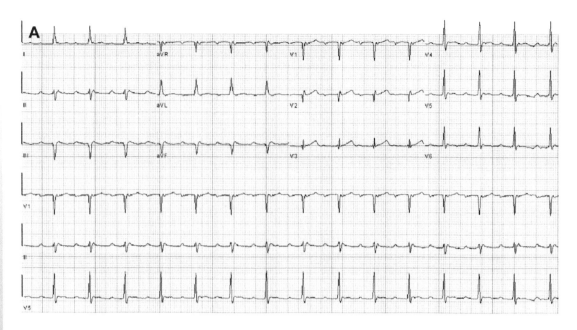

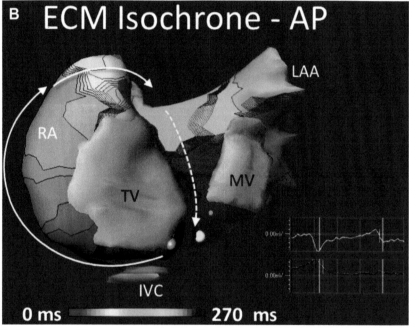

Fig. 5. (*A*) ECG of a 67-year-old man with a previous left atrial myxoma surgery. The ECG shows an atrial tachycardia with P waves in lead V1 resembling normal sinus rhythm morphology with positive component preceding the negative component. There are also positive P waves in inferior leads. This arrhythmia can be from either the left or the right atrium. It could be either focal or reentry. (*B*) The ECM isochronal map identified a reentrant circuit around the tricuspid annulus that represented typical clockwise atrial flutter. About 90% of the CL of the tachycardia is mapped. The recordings of the electrograms from the earliest and latest site in the circuit (head-meets-tail) are also shown. The color of the electrograms corresponds to the color of the dots in the map (*purple and yellow*), representing the sites where these 2 recordings were made. The tachycardia was confirmed during EPS to be cavo-tricuspid-isthmus dependent and was successfully ablated. MV, mitral valve area; RA, right atrium; TV, tricuspid valve area.

postriotomy scar. ECM accurately diagnosed 85% of the macro-reentrant ATs. The diagnostic accuracy of ECM for the cavotricuspid isthmus- and roof-dependent ATs and the postatriotomy scar-related ATs was found to be 100%. Of 5 perimitral ATs, 4 showed no diagnostic pattern because of 2:1 AV conduction with superimposition of the P waves on the preceding QRS complex and T waves, a situation that may easily be mitigated by use of adenosine. In addition, the 4 episodes of perimitral AT that were not diagnosed accurately with ECM had low P wave amplitude secondary to previous extensive ablation. ECM accurately diagnosed all focal tachycardias in the left and right atria. The overall diagnostic accuracy of ECM compared with invasive EP diagnosis as the gold standard was 92% (100% in patients with de novo ablations, and 83% in patients with previous AF ablations). Although the atrial septum could not be visualized with ECM, the system correctly diagnosed the septal origin of 2 episodes of AT by inferring from the pattern of the epicardial exit observed at the anterior interatrial groove. Furthermore, review of the 12-lead ECG of the figures in this report shows that localization of the tachycardia based on the standard ECG would have been difficult because of extensive previous ablation. In summary, ECM was useful in diagnosing accurately all focal tachycardias and all tachycardias in patients with de novo ablations regardless of the mechanism of the arrhythmia. It was also successful in the localization of the tachycardia in 2 patients with septal origin of the AT. ECM could not accurately diagnose 4 of the 5 perimitral (reentrant) AT. It is our understanding from personal communication with the authors of this study (Dr Ashok Shah, 2014) that this diagnostic limitation observed in perimitral AT cases has been overcome today to a considerable extent by improvement made in the vest and amplifiers that lead to the reduction of the acquired noise. In addition, signal averaging tools were incorporated in the current version of this system and new AT mapping algorithm specific to the system-generated maps were developed.

SUMMARY

In this article, we have provided a review in chronologic order of all the noninvasive attempts and systems that exist to map patients with WPW syndrome and atrial arrhythmias. Importantly, we have summarized these efforts, emphasizing their potential benefits, and discussing the current status of noninvasive mapping of AT and WPW syndrome.

At the moment only reports available of noninvasive mapping in patients with WPW syndrome and atrial tachyarrhythmias are those that have used and are using the ECGI/ECM system. Other systems described in the introduction of this article are either no longer in use or their use has not been reported in recent years. We note that as far as atrial tachyarrhythmias and WPW syndrome are concerned, reports using the ECGI/ECM system have come from 3 centers only. These centers are highly experienced in noninvasive and invasive mapping and have dedicated their efforts for many decades to help develop the current system. It remains to be seen what the results would be if prospective, blinded, and multicenter trials were done.

When discussing the merits of the current noninvasive systems, 2 aspects deserve consideration: ability to determine the mechanism of the arrhythmia, the location of the focus or the AACV, and the ability to identify the critical component of the reentrant circuit. We have seen impressive reports of the system being able to identify and locate: right versus left septal ventricular insertion of AACV, epicardial insertion of the AACV, multiple accessory pathways, and characterize atrial arrhythmias in the presence of complex or unusual anatomy. Consequently, in patients with atrial tachyarrhythmias, the system was able to differentiate the mechanism of the arrhythmia and its location in the vast majority of patients studied. All of these are very important and allow for adequate planning and counseling of the patient regarding the risk of the planned procedure. However, one has to mention that invasive EPS still remains the gold standard in determining both the location and the mechanism of the arrhythmias. Most of these patients mapped noninvasively undergo an invasive procedure anyhow. However, based on the noninvasive mapping data, the invasive procedure will likely be more focused, faster, easier, and safer. The location of the AACV or the atrial tachycardia can readily be determined during invasive procedures. Similarly, the ultimate mechanism of the arrhythmia is determined by using the current gold standard—the entrainment maneuvers. We still do not know how successful noninvasive mapping can be in determining the mechanism of an arrhythmia in severely diseased and scarred atria. Noninvasive mapping needs the atrial signals to be of sufficient amplitude, which may be an issue in diseased atria. However, the system can certainly be helpful in patients who have failed previous ablation and in circumstances in which unusual and difficult anatomy is present or expected. Importantly, one has to mention that any potential advantage of this system may come at the expense of increased radiation exposure in cases where CT scan is used to define the cardiac anatomy. As mentioned earlier, we do need many more patients to be studied in as many centers as possible and in a randomized and prospective fashion. We need this because the potential advantages and features of the system appear to be promising.

REFERENCES

1. Evans JW, Erb BD, Brody DA. Comparative proximity and remoteness characteristics of conventional electrocardiographic leads. Am Heart J 1961;61:615–21.
2. Horan LG, Hand RC, Flowers NC, et al. The influence of electrode placement in the reconstruction and analysis of body surface potential maps from limited thoracic arrays. J Electrocardiol 1980;13(4):311–21.
3. Ramanathan C, Ghanem RN, Jia P, et al. Noninvasive electrocardiographic imaging for cardiac electrophysiology and arrhythmia. Nat Med 2004;10(4):422–8. http://dx.doi.org/10.1038/nm1011.
4. Pfeifer B, Hanser F, Seger M, et al. Patient-specific volume conductor modeling for non-invasive imaging of cardiac electrophysiology. Open Med Inform J 2008;2:32–41. http://dx.doi.org/10.2174/1874431100802010032.
5. Denisov AM, Zakharov EV, Kalinin AV, et al. Numerical methods for some inverse problems of heart electrophysiology. Differ Equ 2009;45(7):1034–43.
6. Yamada K, Toyama J, Wada M, et al. Body surface isopotential mapping in Wolff-Parkinson-White syndrome: noninvasive method to determine the localization of the accessory atrioventricular pathway. Am Heart J 1975;90(6):721–34.
7. Iwa T, Magara T. Correlation between localization of accessory conduction pathway and body surface maps in the Wolff-Parkinson-White syndrome. Jpn Circ J 1981;45(10):1192–8.
8. Kamakura S, Shimomura K, Ohe T, et al. The role of initial minimum potentials on body surface maps in predicting the site of accessory pathways in patients with Wolff-Parkinson-White syndrome. Circulation 1986;74(1):89–96.
9. Benson DW, Sterba R, Gallagher JJ, et al. Localization of the site of ventricular preexcitation with body surface maps in patients with Wolff-Parkinson-White syndrome. Circulation 1982;65(6):1259–68.
10. Liebman J, Zeno JA, Olshansky B, et al. Electrocardiographic body surface potential mapping in the Wolff-Parkinson-White syndrome. Noninvasive determination of the ventricular insertion sites of accessory atrioventricular connections. Circulation 1991;83(3):886–901.
11. Guiraudon GM, Klein GJ, Sharma AD, et al. Surgery for Wolff-Parkinson-White syndrome: further experience with an epicardial approach. Circulation 1986;74(3):525–9.
12. Gallagher JJ, Pritchett EL, Sealy WC, et al. The pre-excitation syndromes. Prog Cardiovasc Dis 1978;20(4):285–327.
13. Berger T, Fischer G, Pfeifer B, et al. Single-beat noninvasive imaging of cardiac electrophysiology of ventricular pre-excitation. J Am Coll Cardiol 2006;48(10):2045–52. http://dx.doi.org/10.1016/j.jacc.2006.08.019.
14. Arruda MS, McClelland JH, Wang X, et al. Development and validation of an ECG algorithm for identifying accessory pathway ablation site in Wolff-Parkinson-White syndrome. J Cardiovasc Electrophysiol 1998;9(1):2–12.
15. Cakulev I, Sahadevan J, Arruda M, et al. Confirmation of novel noninvasive high-density electrocardiographic mapping with electrophysiology study: implications for therapy. Circ Arrhythm Electrophysiol 2013;6(1):68–75. http://dx.doi.org/10.1161/CIRCEP.112.975813.
16. Cochet H, Dubois R, Sacher F, et al. Cardiac arrythmias: multimodal assessment integrating body surface ECG mapping into cardiac imaging. Radiology 2014;271(1):239–47. http://dx.doi.org/10.1148/radiol.13131331.
17. SippensGroenewegen A, Peeters HA, Jessurun ER, et al. Body surface mapping during pacing at multiple sites in the human atrium: P-wave morphology of ectopic right atrial activation. Circulation 1998;97(4):369–80.
18. SippensGroenewegen A, Roithinger FX, Peeters HA, et al. Body surface mapping of atrial arrhythmias: atlas of paced P wave integral maps to localize the focal origin of right atrial tachycardia. J Electrocardiol 1998;31(Suppl):85–91.
19. SippensGroenewegen A, Lesh MD, Roithinger FX, et al. Body surface mapping of counterclockwise and clockwise typical atrial flutter: a comparative analysis with endocardial activation sequence mapping. J Am Coll Cardiol 2000;35(5):1276–87.
20. Wang Y, Schuessler RB, Damiano RJ, et al. Noninvasive electrocardiographic imaging (ECGI) of scar-related atypical atrial flutter. Heart Rhythm 2007;4(12):1565–7. http://dx.doi.org/10.1016/j.hrthm.2007.08.019.
21. Shah AJ, Hocini M, Xhaet O, et al. Validation of novel 3-dimensional electrocardiographic mapping of atrial tachycardias by invasive mapping and ablation: a multicenter study. J Am Coll Cardiol 2013;62(10):889–97. http://dx.doi.org/10.1016/j.jacc.2013.03.082.

Noninvasive Mapping to Guide Atrial Fibrillation Ablation

Han S. Lim, MBBS, PhD, Stephan Zellerhoff, MD, Nicolas Derval, MD,
Arnaud Denis, MD, Seigo Yamashita, MD, Benjamin Berte, MD,
Saagar Mahida, MBChB, Darren Hooks, MBChB, Nora Aljefairi, MD,
Ashok J. Shah, MD, Frédéric Sacher, MD, Meleze Hocini, MD,
Pierre Jais, MD, Michel Haissaguerre, MD*

KEYWORDS

- Noninvasive mapping • Atrial fibrillation • Catheter ablation • Localized drivers

KEY POINTS

- Noninvasive mapping overcomes previous obstacles to panoramic atrial fibrillation (AF) mapping and enables biatrial mapping of the underlying mechanisms in AF.
- Localized reentrant and focal drivers are identified with the use of noninvasive mapping and phase mapping algorithms in patients with AF.
- A strategy of driver-based ablation guided by noninvasive mapping yields promising results and minimizes the extent of ablation.
- Future studies will enhance the role of noninvasive mapping to direct personalized therapy to patients with AF.

INTRODUCTION

Atrial fibrillation (AF) is traditionally thought to be maintained by multiple wave fronts that propagate randomly throughout the atria.[1] In paroxysmal AF, the realization of the role of triggers, mainly from the pulmonary veins (PVs), initiating AF has led to the elimination of PV triggers as the cornerstone of AF ablation therapy.[2,3] However, in persistent AF, the elimination of PV triggers alone does not yield similar results, largely because of wider substrate involvement contributing to the maintenance of the arrhythmia. Various mechanisms, such as multiple wavelets, reentry, and focal sources, have been proposed to maintain persistent AF.[1,2,4,5]

Accumulating evidence now suggests that persistent AF may be driven by localized reentrant and focal sources in the atria.[6–10] However, these localized AF drivers prove difficult to detect, because of AF being a dynamic rhythm and the potential spatiotemporal dynamicity of the underlying sources. Previous attempts to map these localized drivers using endocardial single-point or multielectrode catheters and epicardial surgical plaques have been restricted by the inability to simultaneously map different points in the left and right atria, contact issues, and limited surgical access.[7,10,11] Noninvasive mapping overcomes these difficulties by enabling panoramic beat-to-beat mapping of this dynamic rhythm.[9,12] Initial

Disclosure: Drs Haissaguerre, Jais and Hocini are stockholders in and Dr Shah is a paid consultant to CardioInsight Inc., Cleveland, OH, USA. This work was supported through the Investment of the Future grant, ANR-10-IAHU-04, from the government of France through the Agence National de la Recherche.
IHU LIRYC, Electrophysiology and Heart Modeling Institute, Fondation Bordeaux Université, Bordeaux, France
* Corresponding author.
E-mail address: michel.haissaguerre@chu-bordeaux.fr

Card Electrophysiol Clin 7 (2015) 89–98
http://dx.doi.org/10.1016/j.ccep.2014.11.004

studies with ablation guided by noninvasive mapping to identify and target these localized sources have yielded promising results.[8,9,12]

This article discusses the role of noninvasive mapping to guide AF ablation therapy, including the specific methodology of noninvasive mapping to map AF drivers, current experience and clinical results, and future areas of investigation.

METHODOLOGY OF NONINVASIVE MAPPING TO DETECT ATRIAL FIBRILLATION DRIVERS

The use of noninvasive mapping in the atria has been validated in numerous studies. This technique includes noninvasive mapping of focal atrial tachycardias (ATs), macroreentrant ATs, Wolff-Parkinson-White syndrome, and AF.[13–17] Several advances in the approach to body surface mapping have enabled improved precision mapping of the atria. First, noninvasive body surface mapping is based on the principle that the electric cardiac potential generated and its relation to the surrounding torso volume and the body surface follows the Laplace equation.[14] An inverse solution to the forward problem of electrocardiography is therefore applied. This transformation is refined by applying several computational algorithms during this process to suppress potential errors.[14] Second, the patient-specific three-dimensional (3D) atrial geometry is obtained from noncontrast thoracic computed tomography (CT) scan to improve mapping precision. During the CT scan, the exact locations of all the body surface electrodes on the patient's torso are simultaneously acquired. To record body surface potentials, we use a commercially available noninvasive mapping system (ECVue, Cardioinsight Technologies Inc, Cleveland, OH). The body vest consists of 252 electrodes, and is applied to the patient's torso.

Data from the recorded body surface potentials and segmented patient-specific atrial geometry are subsequently combined. Cardiac potentials derived from the body surface potentials are reconstructed during each beat and projected onto the biatrial shell of the patient.[9] To avoid interference from the QRST signal, we select the T-Q segments for analysis. Windows with R-R pauses greater than or equal to 1000 milliseconds during AF are consecutively recorded. In select patients with rapid ventricular rates, diltiazem is administered to slow the ventricular rate in order to provide adequate recording windows. Noninvasive mapping can be performed at the bedside for patients presenting in AF, before entering the electrophysiology laboratory. For patients presenting in sinus rhythm, AF can be induced in the electrophysiology laboratory by rapid atrial pacing. AF drivers are subsequently analyzed after a predetermined waiting period ($\approx$30 minutes in initial studies). During this time, other procedural steps, such as left atrial access and creation of the atrial geometry using an electroanatomic mapping system, may be undertaken.

From the recorded potentials, activation maps and phase maps can both be created for analysis.[11,12] Activation maps are created using the conventional unipolar electrogram intrinsic deflection-based method ($-dV/dT_{max}$ [function of voltage over time]). Filtering processes are applied to remove signal artifacts and to optimize phase transformation.[9,11] Phase maps during AF are created using specific phase mapping algorithms, whereby a representation of the depolarization and repolarization wave fronts are computed from the isophase values corresponding respectively with $\pi/2$ and $-\pi/2$.[12] Videos of the wave propagation patterns during AF are subsequently displayed on the 3D biatrial geometry of each patient.

With the panoramic phase mapping approach described earlier, localized drivers in AF may be identified, which are largely in one of 2 groups: reentrant and focal. Drivers are classified as reentrant (rotor) when a wave is recorded to rotate fully around a functional core on phase progression. The reentrant drivers are confirmed by sequential activation of local unipolar electrograms covering the local cycle length around a pivot point. Drivers are classified as focal when a wave front originates from a focal site with centrifugal activation, which is verified by a QS pattern on unipolar electrograms. To avoid nonphysiologic errors, in some studies drivers are only classified when 2 or more repeated events are recorded.

In our experience, the localized drivers in each patient display certain spatiotemporal characteristics, but tend to recur around the same regions. Hence, a driver-density map is created in each patient by summating all the drivers recorded in each window onto an aggregated map that is projected on the patient's biatrial geometry. This aggregated driver-density map serves as the roadmap for ablation. To classify the distribution of the observed reentrant and focal drivers, the biatrial geometry is divided into several anatomic domains, for example (1) left PVs and left atrial appendage, (2) right PV/posterior interatrial septum, (3) inferoposterior left atrium (LA) and coronary sinus, (4) superior right atrium (RA), (5) inferior RA, (6) anterior LA/roof, and (7) anteroseptal region.

PAROXYSMAL ATRIAL FIBRILLATION

In patients with paroxysmal AF, ectopic beats originating from the PVs are frequently observed as the trigger initiating AF, thus leading to the concept of PV isolation to eliminate these triggers.[2,3] Zellerhoff and colleagues[18] recently investigated 17 consecutive patients with paroxysmal AF using the described noninvasive mapping system (ECVue, Cardioinsight Technologies Inc, Cleveland, OH). These findings were correlated with invasive multielectrode mapping and radiofrequency (RF) ablation was performed according to the roadmap provided by noninvasive mapping with the end point of AF termination.

Demonstration of Pulmonary Vein Triggers and Extra–Pulmonary Vein Sources

The PVs and their respective junctions with the posterior LA harbored localized drivers in nearly 90% of the patients. Apart from displaying AF drivers in these anticipated PV regions, noninvasive panoramic imaging provided further insight into potential AF drivers localized remote from the PVs. In approximately 50% of the patients, non-PV foci and reentry could be recorded outside the PV regions and the neighboring posterior LA. The right atrial appendage (RAA), the inferior LA, the coronary sinus ostium, and the anterior LA could feature such foci and reentrant drivers. Of the observed localized drivers, 74% were reentrant and 26% were focal drivers. An example of a focal and reentrant drivers in paroxysmal AF is shown in **Fig. 1**.

Results of Invasive Mapping and Impact of Radiofrequency Ablation on Atrial Fibrillation Termination

The results of noninvasive panoramic imaging correlated well with invasive mapping: arrhythmogenic regions frequently harbored rapid electrical activity during AF, or were shown after return to sinus rhythm to spontaneously induce AF (12 of 17 patients). RF ablation of these noninvasively identified regions terminated AF reliably, further supporting the results of the mapping: ablation of the PVs terminated AF in 15 of 17 (88%) patients. Only 2 of 17 patients required ablation of non-PV regions identified by noninvasive mapping to terminate AF. This phenomenon may be explained by triggered activity during AF and potentially indicated additional sources that may manifest after PV isolation.[19]

In conclusion, noninvasive AF mapping shows that paroxysmal AF is related to a dynamic interplay of PV foci and ostial reentrant drivers in humans, matching well with experimental results using optical mapping.[20] Moreover, identification of non-PV drivers is feasible and reliable, guiding further RF ablation in selected patients.

PERSISTENT ATRIAL FIBRILLATION
Persistent Atrial Fibrillation Drivers Identified by Noninvasive Mapping

The feasibility of noninvasive mapping to identify underlying AF patterns was shown by Cuculich and colleagues[11] in a cohort of patients with paroxysmal and persistent AF. With the use of activation mapping, diverse AF patterns were observed, which included multiple wavelets, rotors, and focal sources.[11] Locations that were critical to AF maintenance were identified by noninvasive mapping, which responded to catheter ablation.

In a recent study, Haissaguerre and colleagues[12] described the use of noninvasive mapping to guide ablation in patients with persistent AF. In 103 consecutive patients with persistent AF, noninvasive phase maps during AF were acquired, either at the bedside before entering the electrophysiology laboratory or just before ablation. These maps revealed constantly changing dynamic beat-to-beat wave fronts during AF. Approximately 80% of the observed drivers were reentrant and approximately 20% were focal. Driver activity displayed spatiotemporal periodicity and reentrant drivers were observed to meander. However, these reentrant drivers recurred at the same region. Reentrant activity was periodic and not sustained, akin to that described in optical mapping and animal studies.[4,21] For reentrant activity, the median number of continuous rotations was 2.6 (2.3–3.3), whereas an average of 6 events was observed from a focal site.[12] Overall, a median of 4 driver regions has to be targeted per patient. In the entire study cohort, reentrant drivers were commonly located in the right PV/septal region, left PV/left atrial appendage region, left inferior wall/coronary sinus region, and upper RA. However, this distribution varied among individual patients. **Fig. 2** shows a reentrant driver identified by noninvasive mapping in the inferior LA.

Persistent Atrial Fibrillation Drivers, Electrogram Characteristics, and Atrial Fibrosis

Because of the spatiotemporal variability of the AF drivers, identifying them using conventional point-by-point mapping or even with the use of regional multielectrode catheters confers inherent difficulties.[11] Bipolar electrogram characteristics of driver versus nondriver regions detected by noninvasive mapping were compared in a subset of

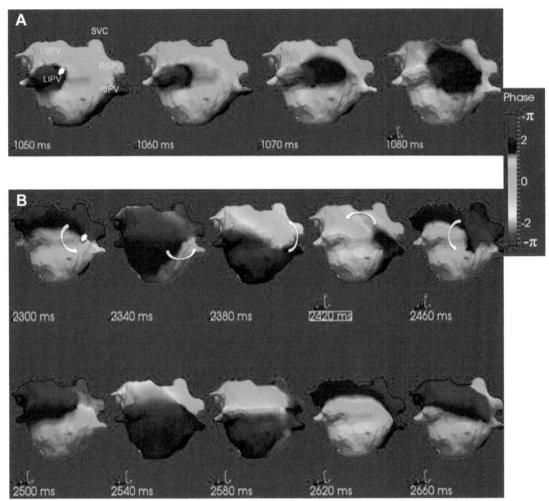

Fig. 1. Phase mapping shows the posterior view of the LA during paroxysmal AF. (*A*) Serial snapshots of a single wave emerging out of the left inferior PV (*white star*) and reaching the right veins in 30 milliseconds while expanding radially to the roof and inferior walls. (*B*) Serial snapshots of 2 successive rotations (*white arrows*) of a rotor located near the ostia of the right veins. The core of the rotor (the white star at the center of the rainbow-colored phases of the rotor) is seen meandering in a small region in this example. The blue wave indicates the depolarizing front, which makes 1 full rotation in 160 milliseconds. The phases of wave propagation are color coded using a rainbow scale. Blue represents the depolarizing wave; green represents the end of repolarization. The wave front can be read by following the blue color. The time (milliseconds) at the bottom of each snapshot represents the moment in the time window when the snapshot was taken. LIPV, left inferior PV; LSPV, left superior PV; RIPV, right inferior PV; RSPV, right superior PV; SVC, superior vena cava. (*From* Haissaguerre M, Hocini M, Shah AJ, et al. Noninvasive panoramic mapping of human atrial fibrillation mechanisms: a feasibility report. J Cardiovasc Electrophysiol 2013;24:713; with permission.)

patients in the study by Haissaguerre and colleagues.[12] Prolonged fractionated electrograms were more commonly found in regions that harbored reentrant AF drivers, conceivably because of local tissue heterogeneity anchoring reentry. In addition, electrograms recorded on a multielectrode catheter covered a large part of the AF cycle length, which is consistent with recordings of localized reentry. At present, studies are underway to further correlate the underlying

diverse AF patterns and drivers revealed by noninvasive mapping with conventional invasive mapping.

There are recent data to indicate that reentrant drivers tend to reside in the patchy zones and border zones of dense fibrosis detected by atrial MRI.[22] In addition, complex fractionated atrial electrograms were found mostly in areas with patchy or no fibrosis, rather than in the densely fibrotic regions.[22] However, although fractionation

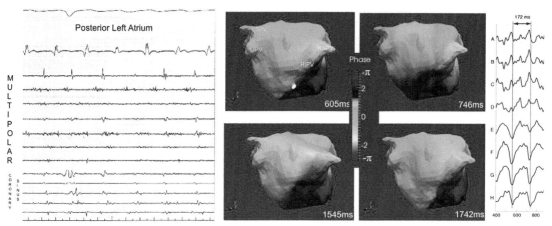

Fig. 2. Intracardiac recordings (*left*), noninvasive phase maps (*middle*), and reconstructed electrograms (*right*) of the posterior LA during persistent AF. The 4 snapshots in the middle show a rotor meandering in the inferior LA at different times. The blue wave indicating the depolarizing front makes a full rotation in 170 to 180 milliseconds. The core of the rotor (the *white star* at the center of the rainbow-colored phases of the rotor) can be seen meandering in a small region. The phases of wave propagation are color coded using a rainbow scale. Blue represents the depolarizing wave; green represents the end of repolarization. The wave front can be read by following the blue color. The time (milliseconds) at the bottom of each snapshot represents the moment in the time window when the snapshot was taken. Right: unipolar electrograms along the path of 1 rotor rotation, before any specific signal processing. Note the varying morphology of electrograms recorded within a small area surrounding the core, and the presence of potentials covering the cycle length (172 milliseconds). (*From* Haissaguerre M, Hocini M, Shah AJ, et al. Noninvasive panoramic mapping of human atrial fibrillation mechanisms: a feasibility report. J Cardiovasc Electrophysiol 2013;24:715; with permission.)

may signal proximity to a driver site, it is not a specific pointer.[23–25] The degree of fractionation may also be influenced by other factors, such as the collision of multiple wave fronts, anisotropic/slow conduction, and adjacent anatomic structures.[26]

Driver-based Catheter Ablation for Persistent Atrial Fibrillation

The optimal ablation approach for these localized drivers is still under investigation. In a recent study, an aggregated driver-density map was created in each individual patient and used as a roadmap to guide catheter ablation.[12] Over a cumulative recording period, specific regions of dense driver activity emerge on the aggregated AF map. The driver regions are then ranked according to overall prevalence of driver activity. Catheter ablation is started at the region of highest driver density, where point-by-point RF lesions are applied at the area covering the reentrant or focal drivers. The local ablation end point at each driver region is local cycle length slowing (**Fig. 3**). Complete abolition of regional electrograms is not required and not pursued, to avoid excessive ablation and potentially arrhythmogenic scar. Each driver region is progressively ablated in a decreasing

order, aiming for the overall procedural end point of AF termination. RF power delivery was set at 30 to 40 W using an irrigated-tip catheter, with a lower setting at the posterior LA wall, and temperature was limited to 45°C.

In the aforementioned study, PV isolation was completed at the end of the procedure during sinus rhythm if required. Should patients remain in AF at the end of the procedure, direct-current cardioversion was performed. In patients in whom AF terminated into AT, these intervening ATs were subsequently ablated.[12] **Figs. 4** and **5** show 2 case examples of patients with persistent AF who underwent driver-guided ablation.

Clinical Outcomes

The median number of targeted driver regions varied with the duration of continuous AF, from 3 regions in AF lasting less than or equal to 3 months to 6 regions in AF lasting greater than or equal to 6 months. Ablation of driver regions alone terminated AF in 75% of patients with early persistent AF, which declined with longer duration of AF (<6 months) up to 13% in long-lasting AF. Approximately two-thirds of these cases terminated into an intermediate AT, whereas approximately one-third terminated directly into sinus rhythm.

Ablation Approach

Driver regions are ablated sequentially based on statistical prevalence

Regional Endpoint:

A) Local cycle length increase beyond appendage cycle length

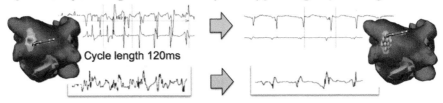

B) Transformation of rapid complex signals into slower simple signals

C) Electrogram abolition is undue/excessive

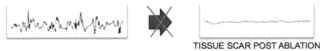

TISSUE SCAR POST ABLATION

Fig. 3. Driver-based ablation approach. The local regional end points are (A) increase in local regional cycle length beyond the appendage cycle length, and (B) transformation of the rapid complex signals into slower simple signals.

During follow-up at 12 months, 64% of patients were in stable sinus rhythm, 22% in AT, and 20% in AF. A repeat procedure was performed in 16 patients: 12 for AT and 4 for AF. Freedom from AF on follow-up was greater in patients with procedural AF termination compared with those without (85% vs 63%; $P = .045$). Compared with a control group of patients who underwent

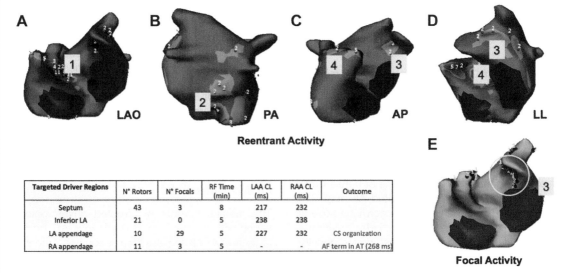

Targeted Driver Regions	N° Rotors	N° Focals	RF Time (min)	LAA CL (ms)	RAA CL (ms)	Outcome
Septum	43	3	8	217	232	
Inferior LA	21	0	5	238	238	
LA appendage	10	29	5	227	232	CS organization
RA appendage	11	3	5	-	-	AF term in AT (268 ms)

Fig. 4. A 68-year-old man with persistent AF of 7 months' duration. The patient was on amiodarone. Baseline AF cycle length was 215 milliseconds. Noninvasive mapping identified 4 driver regions. These driver regions were ablated sequentially, starting from the region of highest density: (1) septum; (2) inferior LA; (3) LA appendage; and (4) RA appendage. Panels A to D show regions of reentrant activity; panel E shows sites of focal activity. Progressive AF cycle length prolongation was observed with the ablation of these drivers, with organization of coronary sinus (CS) activity following the third driver region. AF terminated into AT following ablation of the fourth driver region. Total RF time for driver ablation was 23 minutes. LAA, LA appendage.

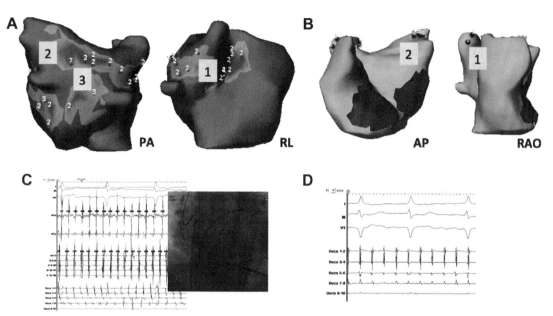

Fig. 5. A 65-year-old man with 7 months of persistent AF. (*A*) The aggregated driver-density map showed reentrant drivers that concentrated around the right PV ostium/septum, the posterior and inferior LA, and the left PV ostium (left panel, posteroanterior [PA] view of the LA and RA; right panel, right lateral [RL] view). (*B*) Aggregated driver-density map of focal drivers originating from the left and right upper PVs (left panel, anteroposterior [AP] view of the LA and RA; right panel, right anterior oblique [RAO] view). (*C*) The mean baseline AF cycle length was 164 milliseconds in the LA and 165 milliseconds in the RA. Inset: the ablation catheter was positioned at the LA appendage and the multispline catheter at the RA appendage. A decapolar catheter was positioned in the coronary sinus. (*D*) AF terminated into AT following ablation of the 3 identified driver regions: (1) right PV/septum, (2) left PV/LA appendage, and (3) inferoposterior LA.

conventional stepwise ablation, driver-guided ablation yielded comparable 12-month clinical outcomes, but the amount of ablation was halved (28 ± 17 minutes vs 65 ± 33 minutes for AF termination).[12] In this regard, an ablation strategy targeting localized drivers has the potential to minimize the extent of ablation and avoid unnecessary damage to atrial tissue.

The utility and feasibility of noninvasive mapping to guide ablation in persistent AF is currently being evaluated in a prospective multicenter study (Noninvasive Mapping of Atrial Fibrillation study [AFACART]).[27] The AFACART study is a prospective multicenter study involving 8 European centers, enrolling patients with persistent AF refractory to more than 1 antiarrhythmic agent undergoing catheter ablation. The study aims to evaluate acute procedural termination rates, RF duration, procedural time, and long-term freedom from persistent AF at 12-months with a noninvasive mapping–guided ablation approach, compared with conventional methods of ablation. At present, 98 patients are enrolled (average age, 64 ± 8 years; average duration of continuous AF, 5.3 ± 5.6 months). In 93% of these cases, driver ablation alone resulted in a significant impact on the AF

process (with either AF cycle length prolongation [in 30%], or AF termination to AT or sinus rhythm [in 63%]).[27] Initial follow-up at 3-months showed only 7% AF recurrence. The initial results from this study indicate that an ablation approach using noninvasive mapping is feasible in centers with minimal or no prior experience.

CURRENT CHALLENGES AND FUTURE AREAS OF INVESTIGATION

Noninvasive mapping for atrial arrhythmias has advanced significantly over the last few years. With the increased density of body surface electrodes in carefully positioned locations on the torso, coupled with knowledge of the precise locations of surface electrodes in relation to the individualized patient atrial geometry, mapping accuracy is improved. However, several challenges remain. First, certain regions remain difficult to image, such as the interatrial septum and the left PV/LA appendage ridge. In such areas, AF propagation patterns need to be verified from multiple angles and by examining the raw electrograms. Drivers arising from the septum typically display a breakout pattern that spreads simultaneously to the left and right atria. Second, with the current signal/noise ratio, the spatial accuracy is ~6 mm and smaller signals less than 0.15 mV may not reliably be detected. This problem may present a challenge in areas of scar or previous ablation. Mapping of global wave front activity is not affected, however a small (subcentimeter) reentrant source may be confused with a focal source as only centrifugal propagation is observed from one region. Third, during transformation of data to a phase-based analysis, potential false-positives of reentrant activity may be recorded because of interpolation of incomplete wave curvatures. To control for this, local raw electrograms need to be verified to show sequential activation around a pivot point, or stricter definitions should be applied, such as greater than or equal to 2 continuous rotations, to increase specificity. In addition, current approaches use noncontrast CT scanning (<2 mSv) to obtain the patient's atrial geometry. Patients undergoing repeat procedures do not require a repeat CT scan, because the previous atrial geometry may be reused. Although the limited amount of radiation is likely to decrease with continuing technological advancements, studies are underway to investigate the use of other imaging modalities such as MRI or rotational angiography to delineate atrial geometry.

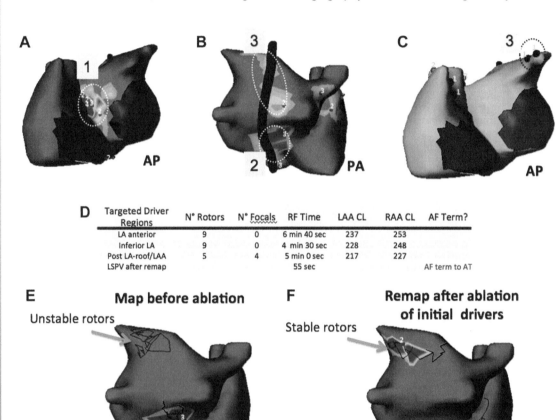

Fig. 6. A 54-year-old man with persistent AF (longest duration, 5 months). The patient was on amiodarone. Baseline AF cycle length was 225 milliseconds in the LA appendage and 243 milliseconds in the RA appendage. Baseline noninvasive mapping revealed 3 reentrant driver regions: (1) anterior LA/anteroseptal region, (2) inferior LA, and (3) posterior LA, with some further unstable reentries extending to the roof/left PV region. (A) AP and (B) PA views, showing CT-based biatrial geometry of the individual patient with reentrant activity marked in orange. (C) Focal activity arising from the LA appendage. The 3 identified driver regions were targeted sequentially: (1) anterior LA/anteroseptal region, (2) inferior LA, and (3) posterior LA-roof/LAA. Total RF time, 16 minutes (D). Noninvasive mapping was repeated thereafter, showing the disappearance of the inferior LA driver (E and F). However, the left superior PV region, which initially showed unstable reentries, now showed more stable driver activity (F). Note that no rapid activity or fractionation was observed at this site. Ablation at this spot (55 seconds of RF) terminated AF into AT, which was slow and irregular and self-terminated within 5 minutes. No further AF was inducible after the last ablation.

Future areas of investigation include the role of remapping during an ablation procedure to identify dynamic changes, such as the successful elimination or emergence of new drivers during ablation. This will enable a further individualized or tailored approach, potentially improving the results (**Fig. 6**). Other areas of study include the role of direct-current cardioversion before ablation to aid in reverse remodeling and its effects on driver-based ablation. The administration of anti-arrhythmic agents and concurrent noninvasive mapping to identify dominant drivers, and the effect of chemical cardioversion following driver-based ablation, are other areas worth investigating. Noninvasive mapping may also serve as a risk-stratifying tool to evaluate the underlying AF processes and extent of electrical remodeling, complementing structural change information obtained from MRI.

SUMMARY

Recent technological advancements have enabled noninvasive mapping to provide unprecedented panoramic beat-to-beat mapping of AF and its underlying dynamic processes. Driver-based ablation guided by noninvasive mapping yields promising clinical results and limits the extent of ablation. Future studies investigating the use of concurrent noninvasive mapping during driver-based ablation and the effect of antiarrhythmics on AF drivers will further enhance the ability to provide a personalized approach to treating AF.

REFERENCES

1. Allessie MA, Lammers WJ, Bonke FI, et al. Experimental evaluation of Moe's multiple wavelet hypothesis of atrial fibrillation. In: Zipes DP, Jalife J, editors. Cardiac arrhythmias. New York: Grune & Stratton; 1985. p. 265–75.
2. Haissaguerre M, Jais P, Shah DC, et al. Spontaneous initiation of atrial fibrillation by ectopic beats originating in the pulmonary veins. N Engl J Med 1998;339:659–66.
3. Calkins H, Kuck KH, Cappato R, et al. 2012 HRS/EHRA/ECAS expert consensus statement on catheter and surgical ablation of atrial fibrillation: recommendations for patient selection, procedural techniques, patient management and follow-up, definitions, endpoints, and research trial design: a report of the Heart Rhythm Society (HRS) Task Force on Catheter and Surgical Ablation of Atrial Fibrillation. Developed in partnership with the European Heart Rhythm Association (EHRA), a registered branch of the European Society of Cardiology (ESC) and the European Cardiac Arrhythmia Society (ECAS); and in collaboration with the American College of Cardiology (ACC), American Heart Association (AHA), the Asia Pacific Heart Rhythm Society (APHRS), and the Society of Thoracic Surgeons (STS). Endorsed by the governing bodies of the American College of Cardiology Foundation, the American Heart Association, the European Cardiac Arrhythmia Society, the European Heart Rhythm Association, the Society of Thoracic Surgeons, the Asia Pacific Heart Rhythm Society, and the Heart Rhythm Society. Heart Rhythm 2012;9:632–96.e21.
4. Skanes AC, Mandapati R, Berenfeld O, et al. Spatiotemporal periodicity during atrial fibrillation in the isolated sheep heart. Circulation 1998;98:1236–48.
5. Sanders P, Berenfeld O, Hocini M, et al. Spectral analysis identifies sites of high-frequency activity maintaining atrial fibrillation in humans. Circulation 2005;112:789–97.
6. Schuessler RB, Grayson TM, Bromberg BI, et al. Cholinergically mediated tachyarrhythmias induced by a single extrastimulus in the isolated canine right atrium. Circ Res 1992;71:1254–67.
7. Sahadevan J, Ryu K, Peltz L, et al. Epicardial mapping of chronic atrial fibrillation in patients: preliminary observations. Circulation 2004;110:3293–9.
8. Narayan SM, Krummen DE, Shivkumar K, et al. Treatment of atrial fibrillation by the ablation of localized sources: CONFIRM (Conventional Ablation for Atrial Fibrillation With or Without Focal Impulse and Rotor Modulation) trial. J Am Coll Cardiol 2012;60: 628–36.
9. Haissaguerre M, Hocini M, Shah AJ, et al. Noninvasive panoramic mapping of human atrial fibrillation mechanisms: a feasibility report. J Cardiovasc Electrophysiol 2013;24:711–7.
10. Haissaguerre M, Hocini M, Sanders P, et al. Localized sources maintaining atrial fibrillation organized by prior ablation. Circulation 2006;113:616–25.
11. Cuculich PS, Wang Y, Lindsay BD, et al. Noninvasive characterization of epicardial activation in humans with diverse atrial fibrillation patterns. Circulation 2010;122:1364–72.
12. Haissaguerre M, Hocini M, Denis A, et al. Driver domains in persistent atrial fibrillation. Circulation 2014;130:530–8.
13. Shah AJ, Hocini M, Xhaet O, et al. Validation of novel 3-dimensional electrocardiographic mapping of atrial tachycardias by invasive mapping and ablation: a multicenter study. J Am Coll Cardiol 2013;62: 889–97.
14. Rudy Y. Noninvasive electrocardiographic imaging of arrhythmogenic substrates in humans. Circ Res 2013;112:863–74.
15. Wang Y, Cuculich PS, Woodard PK, et al. Focal atrial tachycardia after pulmonary vein isolation: noninvasive mapping with electrocardiographic imaging (ECGI). Heart Rhythm 2007;4:1081–4.

16. Wang Y, Schuessler RB, Damiano RJ, et al. Non-invasive electrocardiographic imaging (ECGI) of scar-related atypical atrial flutter. Heart Rhythm 2007;4:1565–7.

17. Ghosh S, Rhee EK, Avari JN, et al. Cardiac memory in patients with Wolff-Parkinson-White syndrome: noninvasive imaging of activation and repolarization before and after catheter ablation. Circulation 2008; 118:907–15.

18. Zellerhoff S, Hocini M, Dubois R, et al. Mechanisms driving paroxysmal AF displayed by noninvasive panoramic imaging (AB 35-05). Heart Rhythm 2013;10:S41–95.

19. Takahashi Y, Hocini M, O'Neill MD, et al. Sites of focal atrial activity characterized by endocardial mapping during atrial fibrillation. J Am Coll Cardiol 2006;47:2005–12.

20. Jalife J, Berenfeld O, Mansour M. Mother rotors and fibrillatory conduction: a mechanism of atrial fibrillation. Cardiovasc Res 2002;54:204–16.

21. Ryu K, Shroff SC, Sahadevan J, et al. Mapping of atrial activation during sustained atrial fibrillation in dogs with rapid ventricular pacing induced heart failure: evidence for a role of driver regions. J Cardiovasc Electrophysiol 2005;16:1348–58.

22. Jadidi AS, Cochet H, Shah AJ, et al. Inverse relationship between fractionated electrograms and atrial fibrosis in persistent atrial fibrillation: combined magnetic resonance imaging and high-density mapping. J Am Coll Cardiol 2013;62:802–12.

23. Konings KT, Smeets JL, Penn OC, et al. Configuration of unipolar atrial electrograms during electrically induced atrial fibrillation in humans. Circulation 1997;95:1231–41.

24. Narayan SM, Shivkumar K, Krummen DE, et al. Panoramic electrophysiological mapping but not electrogram morphology identifies stable sources for human atrial fibrillation: stable atrial fibrillation rotors and focal sources relate poorly to fractionated electrograms. Circ Arrhythm Electrophysiol 2013;6: 58–67.

25. Zlochiver S, Yamazaki M, Kalifa J, et al. Rotor meandering contributes to irregularity in electrograms during atrial fibrillation. Heart Rhythm 2008; 5:846–54.

26. Lim HS, Haissaguerre M. Focused review: mapping human atrial fibrillation to guide catheter ablation. In: Bonow RO, Mann DL, Zipes DP, et al, editors. Braunwald's heart disease: a textbook of cardiovascular medicine. 9th edition. Philadelphia: Saunders/Elsevier; 2013 (digital edition).

27. Knecht S, Rostock T, Arentz T, et al. Successful ablation of persistent AF based on a non-invasive mapping to identify drivers: the AFACART multicenter study. Heart Rhythm 2014;11(Suppl 5):135, 1–145.

Noninvasive Mapping of Ventricular Arrhythmias

 CrossMark

Ashok J. Shah, MD*, Han S. Lim, MBBS, PhD, Seigo Yamashita, MD,
Stephan Zellerhoff, MD, Benjamin Berte, MD, Saagar Mahida, MBChB,
Darren Hooks, MBChB, Nora Aljefairi, MD, Nicolas Derval, MD, Arnaud Denis, MD,
Frédéric Sacher, MD, Pierre Jais, MD, Rémi Dubois, PhD, Meleze Hocini, MD,
Michel Haissaguerre, MD

KEYWORDS

- Noninvasive mapping • Ventricular arrhythmias • Ventricual premature beat
- Ventricular tachycardia • Electrical scar • Arrhythmogenic substrate

KEY POINTS

- As validated by electrophysiologic studies, noninvasive electrocardiographic mapping can be undertaken preprocedurally and periprocedurally to accurately diagnose the mechanism of ventricular arrhythmia (focal vs reentrant), identify the chamber of interest, and localize the site of focal arrhythmia.
- Such prior information, which is superior to that obtained from the conventional 12-lead ECG, provides necessary guidance to facilitate catheter ablation in index and previously failed procedures.
- Noninvasive mapping has demonstrated the ability to image arrhythmogenic ventricular substrate having electrophysiologic characteristics of low voltage, altered sinus rhythm activation, electrogram fragmentation, and presence of late potentials in postinfarction myocardium, which correlated well with the anatomic location of scar as depicted by MRI and radionuclide scan.
- Although spatial accuracy of noninvasive imaging has been cited as a possible limitation, the most intriguing aspect of ventricular imaging involves the variable contributions of the endocardium and epicardium to the arrhythmic activity and its inability to directly visualize the interventricular septum.

INTRODUCTION

For more than 100 years, 12-lead electrocardiography (ECG) has been the standard-of-care tool, which involves measuring electrical potentials from limited sites on the body surface to diagnose cardiac disorder, its possible mechanism, and the likely site of origin. Several decades of research has led to the development of a 252-lead ECG-based three-dimensional imaging modality to refine noninvasive diagnosis and improve the management of heart rhythm disorders.[1] This article reviews the clinical potential of this noninvasive mapping technique in identifying the sources of electrical disorders and guiding the catheter ablation of ventricular arrhythmias (premature ventricular beats and ventricular tachycardia [VT]). We also briefly refer to the noninvasive electrical imaging of the arrhythmogenic ventricular substrate based on the electrophysiologic characteristics of postinfarction ventricular myocardium.

Disclosure: This work was supported through the Investment of the Future grant, ANR-10-IAHU-04, from the government of France through the Agence National de la Recherche.

IHU LIRYC, Electrophysiology and Heart Modeling Institute, Fondation Bordeaux Université, Bordeaux, France

* Corresponding author. Service du Pr Haissaguerre, Department of Rhythmologie, Hôpital Cardiologique du Haut-Lévêque, Avenue de Magellan, Pessac, Bordeaux 33604, France.

E-mail address: drashahep@gmail.com

Card Electrophysiol Clin 7 (2015) 99–107
http://dx.doi.org/10.1016/j.ccep.2014.11.014

MAPPING TECHNIQUE

The signal acquisition from the patient and subsequent computational methods used in the reconstruction of noninvasive maps using multiple torso electrodes have been previously described.[1] Briefly, a 252-electrode vest is applied to the patient's torso and connected to the noninvasive imaging system and surface potentials are recorded. It is followed by a noncontrast thoracic computed tomography (CT) scan to obtain high-resolution images of the heart and the vest electrodes. The three-dimensional epicardial biventricular geometry is reconstructed from segmental CT images. The relative positions of body surface electrodes can be visualized on the torso geometry. The system reconstructs epicardial potentials, unipolar electrograms, and activation maps from torso potentials during each beat/cycle using mathematical reconstruction algorithms. Details of the mathematical methods have been provided in detail elsewhere.[2–6]

VENTRICULAR PREMATURE COMPLEX AND TACHYCARDIA

Premature ventricular complexes (PVCs) or outflow tract (OT) VTs are commonly encountered in clinical practice.[7] Localizing the origin of these arrhythmias can be challenging and it may be further complicated in cases where they occur infrequently or last transiently (ie, few beats). Noninvasive mapping is particularly useful in diagnosing the mechanism of arrhythmia (focal vs reentrant), identifying the chamber of interest, and localizing the site of focal arrhythmia.[7,8] In

animal models, the cardiac activation sequences during single or multipoint pacing and VT are accurately depicted by noninvasive mapping.[9] The origin of focal firing and activation sequence of polymorphic VT, such as torsades de pointes, can also be identified noninvasively.[10] The clinical use of noninvasive mapping in reentrant and focal ventricular arrhythmias including the PVCs has been validated by invasive electrophysiologic studies (EPS) and ablation.[7,11]

Intini and colleagues[12] used the electrocardiomapping (ECM) technique for the first time in a clinical setting to guide diagnosis and therapy for a focal VT in a young athlete. Isolated ventricular ectopic beats of an identical morphology to the sustained tachycardia were mapped before the invasive procedure and their origin was localized to the left ventricular (LV) apical diverticulum. Importantly, the QS wave pattern of the reconstructed electrogram from the site of origin of the ectopies indicated that those beats were emanating from the ventricular epicardium at that site. **Fig. 1** shows a clinical example of such a ventricular beat. In the electrophysiology laboratory, the sustained tachycardia was induced in the presence of isoproterenol. Intracardiac activation mapping during tachycardia demonstrated earliest activation in the apical LV diverticulum. During sinus rhythm, pace map at that site was remarkably similar to the tachycardia morphology in 12/12 ECG leads. Electroanatomic three-dimensional mapping of the LV chamber performed during the ectopy also identified the earliest site of activation at the LV apex in the region of the diverticulum, consistent with a focal origin of the tachycardia. Later, transient

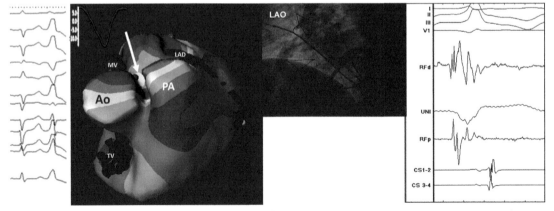

Fig. 1. Biventricular isopotential map (*yellow* denotes the earliest activation) during premature ventricular complex (12-lead ECG). Inserted is an epicardial virtual electrogram (QS morphology) from the earliest site. Also shown are the local intracardiac electrograms at the same site before the start of successful ablation. Ao, aortic root; LAD, left anterior descending artery; LAO, left anterior oblique; MV, mitral valve; PA, pulmonary artery; TV, tricuspid valve.

resolution of the tachycardia during several radio-frequency applications delivered endocardially to the area supported an epicardial origin for the arrhythmia. On invasive epicardial approach, the earliest activation of the ventricular ectopy was identified in a region of low voltage at the LV apex overlying the region of endocardial abnormality. Cryolesions (-70°C) were placed in the low-voltage area. Close proximity to the phrenic nerve, assessed by capture during pacing, precluded complete ablation of the region resulting in recurrence of the arrhythmia.

Wang and colleagues[13] noninvasively obtained information on the site of initiation, VT mechanism (focal or reentrant), and depth of VT origin (epicardial, mid-myocardial, or endocardial). The study examined 26 ventricular arrhythmias in 25 patients (tachycardias [N = 9], premature beats) before (N = 19) and during (N = 4) the invasive procedure. Noninvasive electrocardiographic imaging (ECGI) was in agreement with invasive electrophysiologic study in 10 out of 11 right ventricular (RV) sites (91%) and in 11 out of 12 LV sites (92%). For the two patients with discrepancies between invasive and noninvasive modalities, the discrepant locations were in proximity to each other. For the patient with right posteroseptal RV location, ECGI imaged the right posterolateral base as the location. This patient had undergone previous ablations of a right posteroseptal accessory pathway and a right atriofascicular pathway in the posterolateral base, which were suspected to have played roles in the discrepancy between the two diagnoses. For the patient with apical LV location, ECGI imaged the mid-anterior LV as the location. This patient had a large LV apical aneurysm and several different VT morphologies with discrepancy possibly from the comparison of two different VTs sequentially imaged noninvasively followed by invasively. The arrhythmia mechanism was correctly diagnosed as focal (18 out of 18) and reentrant (five out of five) in 100% of patients based on the centrifugal and early meeting–late patterns of activation, respectively. Furthermore, invasive findings were compared with ECG imaging for determining epicardial versus nonepicardial locations of VT. Because of the thin tissue in the OT, patients with OT were excluded. Of the 13 remaining patients, the invasive study determined the location to be endocardial in six, epicardial in five, and mid-myocardial in two. All five patients with epicardial location had a QS wave at the site of earliest activation (100%), indicative of epicardial origin, noninvasively. Among the patients with a nonepicardial location, the local electrogram at the earliest site demonstrated a small r wave in seven of eight (88%).

Similarly, Cakulev and colleagues[11] undertook noninvasive ECM in 27 patients with varied arrhythmias wherein three-dimensional epicardial activation maps were generated from greater than 250 body surface electrograms using heart-torso geometry obtained from CT images. ECM activation maps were compared with standard 12-lead ECG diagnoses, and confirmed with invasive EPS. Among 27 patients, 10 patients had been diagnosed with clinically relevant PVCs and 1 had sustained exercise-induced VT. Of 10 patients with symptomatic PVCs, 6 originated from the right or left ventricular outflow tract area (RVOT, LVOT). ECM accurately localized the ventricular chamber of origin and the earliest site of activation in four out of six patients. A representative example is shown in **Fig. 2**. Of the two patients with PVCs in whom ECM was not successfully confirmed with EPS, one had PVCs that were transiently suppressed with radiofrequency ablation of the posteroseptal area of the RVOT at the site of a previously repaired ventricular septal defect. In the other, again, only transient suppression of the PVCs was seen during delivery of radiofrequency energy in the LVOT. In both patients, transient suppression of the PVCs during ablation was seen at the sites of earliest onset of electric activation predicted by ECM. This may not indicate ECM inaccuracy, but rather could represent a problem with delivering adequate radiofrequency energy at the site correctly identified by invasive EPS and ECM. Alternatively, both the invasive EPS and ECM maps, although concordant, failed to identify the correct location. In one patient who had an epicardial origin of PVCs, ECM was able to identify the epicardial origin, confirmed by the distinct QS complex morphology of the electrogram at earliest site of activation (**Fig. 3**).

ECM was also able to deduce the origin of the PVCs in one patient who had two simultaneous epicardial breakthroughs. In this patient, two simultaneous, but disparate, epicardial breakthroughs were observed in both ventricles. Some of the breakthroughs consistently coincided with the same location of normal epicardial breakthroughs during sinus rhythm. This supported the diagnosis that the PVCs originated from the His-Purkinje system, and that both the left and right ventricles were involved. A representative image of this example with detailed explanation is shown in **Fig. 4**. This type of diagnosis would have been much more difficult to deduce with conventional endocardial activation mapping. In the patient with exercise-induced, sustained VT, ECM accurately identified the focal origin of tachycardia in the LVOT, where the arrhythmia was ultimately successfully ablated between the right and left

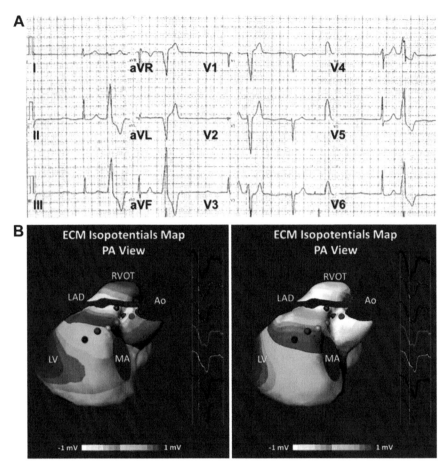

Fig. 2. (*A*) The 12-lead ECG of a 44-year-old man with a previously failed RVOT ablation in the right ventricle. The PVC morphology shows a late transition between V3 and V4. The limb leads display an inferior axis, with the QRS complex being positive in lead I and negative in lead AVL. This would likely place the origin of the PVC in the RVOT, but off the ventricular septum or in the posterior ventricular septum. Because of the late transition on the ECG, the PVC would not be expected to originate on the LV side. (*B*) Two isopotential maps from the ECM show the propagation of the depolarizing wavefront. The *left* shows the location of the earliest activation of the PVC in the vicinity of the proximal left anterior descending coronary artery, but on the left side of the ventricular septum. The site of the earliest depolarization is in *white*. In both panels of *B*, on the right side of the map, the electrograms with a QS complex morphology are shown, indicating epicardial origin. The electrograms around, but not at, the focus lack the sharp negative deflection of the focal electrogram and exhibit more slurring of the downslope. The *vertical lines* across the electrograms show the time point at which the potential was measured. The PVC was accurately mapped to this location during the invasive electrophysiologic study. Ao, aortic root; LAD, left anterior descending artery; MA, mitral annulus; PA, posteroanterior. (*From* Cakulev I, Sahadevan J, Arruda M, et al. Confirmation of novel noninvasive high-density electrocardiographic mapping with electrophysiology study: implications for therapy. Circ Arrhythm Electrophysiol 2013;6:71; with permission.)

coronary cusps. It also accurately identified the focal mechanism of this tachycardia. Two patients had PVCs originating from the LV free wall and ECM accurately predicted the site of the earliest activation.

In a recently published work of Jamil-Copley and colleagues,[7] where the investigators used the same noninvasive mapping technique as Cakulev and colleagues,[11] patients wore a body vest consisting of 252 surface electrodes for

noninvasive localization of clinically symptomatic ventricular OT arrhythmias. Patients were allowed to ambulate and the vest was applied up to 5 hours before the procedure to capture the culprit arrhythmia. Cardiac potentials, activation maps, and voltage maps were derived from noninvasive mapping.

There were 24 patients (eight men; mean age, 50 ± 18 years) with one clinical VT/PVC each (23 with left bundle branch block morphology) in the

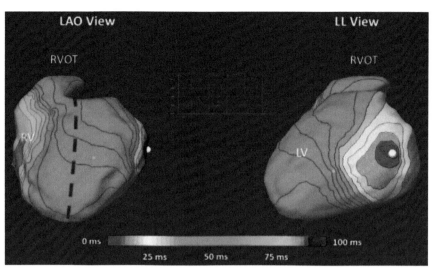

Fig. 3. Activation sequence obtained by electrocardiographic mapping (ECM) of a premature ventricular complex originating from the epicardial surface of the left ventricle. A color-coded scale with a range from 0 to 100 milliseconds is provided for comparison. Left anterior oblique (LAO) and left lateral (LL) views of the cardiac activation sequence are represented. The earliest site of activation is represented with a *yellow dot*. The electrogram recording from that site shows a typical QS complex morphology identified by *arrows* indicating the earliest initial activation in the epicardium. RV, right ventricle; RVOT, right ventricular outflow tract. (*From* Cakulev I, Sahadevan J, Arruda M, et al. Confirmation of novel noninvasive high-density electrocardiographic mapping with electrophysiology study: implications for therapy. Circ Arrhythm Electrophysiol 2013;6:71; with permission.)

study. Six patients had previously undergone EPS, three having had unsuccessful ablation. One patient with recurrent symptoms had undergone four attempts at ablation, but on each previous occasion, ablation could not be completed because of lack of spontaneous clinical ectopy. In 21 of 24 patients with spontaneous PVC/VT preprocedurally, the PVC origins could be mapped and located on the ECM-derived geometry before EPS. In the remaining three patients, ECM located the PVC origin periprocedurally. In all but one patient, PVCs occurred spontaneously or with the initiation of isoproterenol infusion. In only one patient was programmed ventricular stimulation useful for PVC induction. The first ablation lesion was delivered at the site identified by preprocedural/periprocedural ECM, which resulted in acute procedural success in 23 of 24 patients. The local bipolar electrogram at these sites during clinical ectopy preceded QRS onset by 29 ± 9 milliseconds (range, 10–45 milliseconds). At 22 of 24 sites, a 12/12 pace match was achieved. The best pace map at the remaining two sites was 11/12 and 10/12. The mean number of ablation lesions, including consolidation lesions, was 7.5 ± 7 before PVC quiescence. ECM failed to identify the appropriate site of ablation in a single case, where the origin of a left bundle branch block PVC with QRS transition at lead V3/V4 was localized by the ECM to the

RVOT. However, at this site, His bundle capture was noted with an 11/12 ECG pace-map match and local activation, which preceded QRS onset by 40 milliseconds. Ablation was commenced at low-power settings and was stopped early because of the occurrence of a single nonconducted sinus beat. Pacing in the surrounding RVOT region did not reproduce the clinical PVC ECM activation map, which led to exploration of the LVOT. ECM maps created in the LVOT identified a perfect match at the region between the right coronary cusp and the noncoronary cusp with an early local electrogram (−45 milliseconds) and a 12/12 pace-map match. Fluoroscopically this site was anatomically adjacent to the RVOT site explored earlier. Acute procedural success was achieved in all patients after ablation at 18 right and 6 left ventricular sites: three posteroseptal RVOT, eight anteroseptal RVOT, four midseptal RVOT, two posterolateral RVOT, four left coronary cusp, one noncoronary cusp/right coronary cusp junction, and two aortomitral continuity sites. The mean power delivered was 37 ± 13 W.[7]

Erkapic and colleagues[14] undertook randomized clinical comparison between conventional invasive mapping and noninvasive ECM-guided ablation of PVCs, which has been covered in detail elsewhere in this issue.

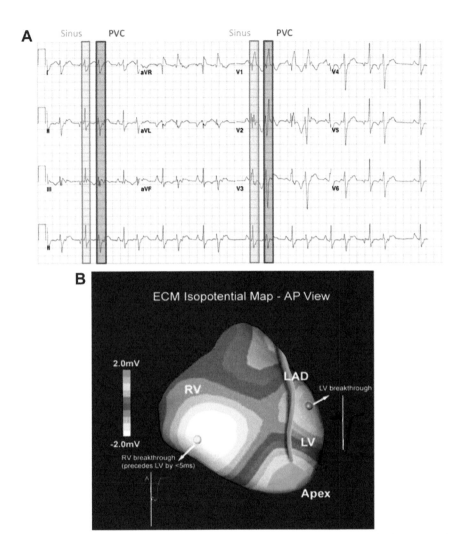

Fig. 4. (*A*) 12-lead ECG of a 22-year-old woman with multiple, symptomatic PVCs. She had a previously failed ablation in the RV free wall. In the *blue highlighted beats* the normal sinus rhythm beat with right bundle-branch block (RBBB) morphology and a normal axis is shown. In the *red highlighted beats* shown is the morphology of the PVC. The morphology is very similar to that of the intrinsic normal sinus beat, because it also has an RBBB morphology, an almost identical QRS complex width, but a slightly different axis. (*B*) Interestingly, the ECM map shows that the PVC has two simultaneous breakthroughs. The *yellow dots* and *pink dots* in the RV and LV, correspondingly, represent the areas with the most negative potential measured by ECM, and are the sites of the earliest depolarization. The *interrupted white dashed line* represents the ventricular septum. At the same time the RV and LV were activated. The right ventricular breakthrough preceded the left by 5 millisec-onds. A correlation with the ECM map during the sinus rhythm map was made, and shows that on the right side, the site of the PVC breakthrough was almost identical to the site of the native sinus rhythm breakthrough, whereas on the left side, they were 7.5 cm apart. Two simultaneous breakthroughs with similar activation patterns as during sinus rhythm suggested an origin of the PVC that invades the His-Purkinje system and activates the RV and LV simultaneously. This would also explain the similar PVC morphology to the intrinsic QRS complex. The recordings of the electrograms from the earliest sites in the RV and LV are also shown. Mapping confirmed the earliest PVC activation to be high in the septum. AP, anteroposterior; LAD, left anterior descending artery. (*From* Cakulev I, Sahadevan J, Arruda M, et al. Confirmation of novel noninvasive high-density electrocardiographic mapping with electrophysiology study: implications for therapy. Circ Arrhythm Electrophysiol 2013;6:72; with permission.)

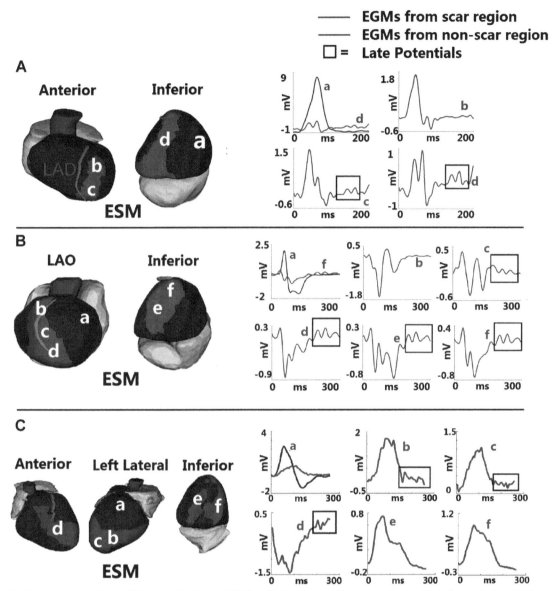

Fig. 5. Late potentials within electrical scar. (*A*) Electrical scar map from a patient with inferoapical scar. Three electrograms (EGMs) from the scar are shown on the right (b–d; *red*). Scar electrogram d is also shown together with nonscar electrogram a (*blue*) in the *upper left*, to highlight differences. Electrograms c and d demonstrate late deflections ("late potentials"; *box*). Late potentials were observed almost exclusively within electrical scar. However (EGM b), late potentials were not present in all scar regions. (*B*) Anteroapical infarct. Late potentials are present in electrograms from inferior and apical regions (c–f), but not the anterior region (b). (*C*) Complex anterior, apical, and inferior infarction. Late potentials are present in several electrograms from the anterior and apical regions (b–d), but not the inferior region (e and f). (*From* Cuculich PS, Zhang J, Wang Y, et al. The electrophysiological cardiac ventricular substrate in patients after myocardial infarction: noninvasive characterization with electrocardiographic imaging. J Am Coll Cardiol 2011;58:1900; with permission.)

In another multicenter study,[15] 35 premature ventricular beats imaged noninvasively were accurately diagnosed in 100% of patients with regard to chamber identification and focal mechanism.

ARRHYTHMOGENIC VENTRICULAR SUBSTRATE

Cuculich and colleagues[16] reported the use of a noninvasive mapping system comprising of 256 surface electrodes and CT-derived chamber

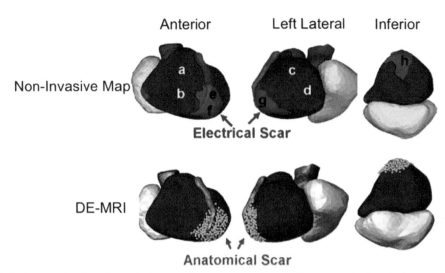

Fig. 6. Clinical example showing relationship between noninvasively mapped electrical scar and delayed enhancement MRI derived anatomic scar in three different projections. a, b, c, d, normal myocardium; e, f, g, h, electrical scar. (*Adapted from* Cucilich PS, Zhang J, Wang Y, et al. The electrophysiological cardiac ventricular substrate in patients after myocardial infarction: noninvasive characterization with electrocardiographic imaging. J Am Coll Cardiol 2011;58:1897; with permission.)

geometry to characterize arrhythmogenic ventricular substrate in 24 patients (mean age, 62 years; mean LV ejection fraction, 30%) postmyocardial infarction. Ventricular substrate for VT was identified noninvasively by low-voltage amplitude (low-voltage regions and very low-voltage regions were defined by electrograms with amplitudes <30% and 15% of the individual's maximum voltage, respectively), fractionated signals (≥2 deflections), late potentials (deflections above the ambient electrical noise level that occurred after the surface QRS), and altered sinus rhythm activation patterns (lines of block, slow conduction/delayed activation) (**Fig. 5**). These maps of electrical substrate were correlated with that of the anatomic substrate obtained using imaging modalities (delayed enhancement MRI for patients without cardiac devices, and myocardial perfusion imaging with single-photon emission CT for patients with cardiac devices).[16] The investigators found that the reconstructed epicardial electrograms displayed the characteristics of reduced amplitude (low voltage) and fractionation. Noninvasive modality colocalized the epicardial electrical scar to the anatomic scar with a high degree of accuracy (sensitivity 89%, specificity 85%) (**Fig. 6**). Sinus rhythm activation patterns were altered by the presence of myocardial scar. Late potentials could be identified and were almost always within ventricular scar. The study concluded that noninvasive mapping can accurately identify the areas of anatomic scar and complements standard anatomic imaging by providing scar-related electrophysiologic characteristics of low voltages, altered sinus rhythm activation, electrogram fragmentation, and presence of late potentials.

LIMITATIONS

Although spatial accuracy of noninvasive imaging has been cited as a possible limitation, the most intriguing aspect of ventricular imaging involves the variable contributions of the endocardium and epicardium to the arrhythmic activity and its inability to directly visualize the interventricular septum. The earliest epicardial activation of VT may not accurately identify the location of an endocardial circuit. Also, slow, discontinuous, delayed systolic or diastolic conduction inside the scar (late potential) may not be easy to visualize especially during the formation of T wave (depolarization activity) and in the presence of contaminating electrical noise.

SUMMARY

Noninvasive ECM can be undertaken preprocedurally and periprocedurally to accurately diagnose the mechanism of ventricular arrhythmia (focal vs reentrant), identify the chamber of interest, and localize the site of focal arrhythmia. This has been validated by EPS. Such prior information, which is superior to that obtained from the conventional 12-lead ECG, provides necessary guidance to facilitate catheter ablation in index and previously failed procedures. The technique has an additional ability to noninvasively image substrate having arrhythmogenic electrophysiologic characteristics in postinfarction myocardium, albeit with some limitations.

REFERENCES

1. Oster HS, Taccardi B, Lux RL, et al. Noninvasive electrocardiographic imaging: reconstruction of epicardial potentials, electrograms, and isochrones and localization of single and multiple electrocardiac events. Circulation 1997;96:1012–24.
2. Tikhonov AN, Arsenin VY. Solutions of ill-posed problems. New York: Wiley; 1977.
3. Calvetti D, Lewis B, Reichel L. GMRES, L-Curves, and Discrete Ill-Posed Problems. BIT 2002;42:44–65.
4. Rudy Y, Oster HS. The electrocardiographic inverse problem. Crit Rev Biomed Eng 1992;20:25–45.
5. Rudy Y, Burnes JE. Noninvasive Electrocardiographic Imaging (ECGI). Ann Noninvasive Electrocardiol 1999;4:340–58, 29.
6. Ramanathan C, Jia P, Ghanem RN, et al. Noninvasive electrocardiographic imaging (ECGI): application of the generalized minimal residual (GMRes) method. Ann Biomed Eng 2003;31:981–94.
7. Jamil-Copley S, Bokan R, Kojodjojo P, et al. Noninvasive electrocardiographic mapping to guide ablation of outflow tract ventricular arrhythmias. Heart Rhythm 2014;11:587–94.
8. Lai D, Sun J, Li Y, et al. Usefulness of ventricular endocardial electric reconstruction from body surface potential maps to noninvasively localize ventricular ectopic activity in patients. Phys Med Biol 2013;58:3897–909.
9. Han C, Pogwizd SM, Killingsworth CR, et al. Noninvasive imaging of three-dimensional cardiac activation sequence during pacing and ventricular tachycardia. Heart Rhythm 2011;8:1266–72.
10. Han C, Pogwizd SM, Killingsworth CR, et al. Noninvasive cardiac activation imaging of ventricular arrhythmias during drug-induced QT prolongation in the rabbit heart. Heart Rhythm 2013;10:1509–15.
11. Cakulev I, Sahadevan J, Arruda M, et al. Confirmation of novel noninvasive high-density electrocardiographic mapping with electrophysiology study: implications for therapy. Circ Arrhythm Electrophysiol 2013;6:68–75.
12. Intini A, Goldstein RN, Jia P, et al. Electrocardiographic imaging (ECGI), a novel diagnostic modality used for mapping of focal left ventricular tachycardia in a young athlete. Heart Rhythm 2005;2(11):1250–2.
13. Wang Y, Cuculich PS, Zhang J, et al. Noninvasive electroanatomic mapping of human ventricular arrhythmias with electrocardiographic imaging. Sci Transl Med 2011;3:98ra84.
14. Erkapic D, Greiss H, Pajitnev D, et al. Clinical impact of a novel three-dimensional electrocardiographic imaging for non-invasive mapping of ventricular arrhythmias: a prospective randomized trial. Europace 2014. [Epub ahead of print].
15. Lindsay B, Varma N, Tchou P, et al. Clinical validation of noninvasive electrocardiographic mapping (ECM) of arrhythmias: a multi-center experience. Heart Rhythm 2012;9(5):S1.
16. Cuculich PS, Zhang J, Wang Y, et al. The electrophysiological cardiac ventricular substrate in patients after myocardial infarction: noninvasive characterization with electrocardiographic imaging. J Am Coll Cardiol 2011;58:1893–902.

Ablation of Premature Ventricular Complexes Exclusively Guided by Three-Dimensional Noninvasive Mapping

Damir Erkapic, MD[a], Thomas Neumann, MD[b],*

KEYWORDS

- Ablation • Ventricular arrhythmia • Premature ventricular contraction
- Electrocardiographic mapping • Noninvasive three-dimensional mapping • ECVUE

KEY POINTS

- ECVUE performance is superior to that of the body surface ECG in premature ventricular complex (PVC) mapping.
- Current data demonstrate that accurate preprocedural PVC localization is responsible for increased ablation procedure efficacy resulting in fewer RF applications required to terminate PVCs, decreased time to first RF application, and decreased total procedure time.
- ECVUE increased patient radiation exposure caused by the requisite CT scan.

INTRODUCTION

The prevalence of idiopathic premature ventricular complexes (PVCs) is reported to be as high as 2.2% in otherwise normal individuals.[1] Alarmingly, increased PVC burden in structurally normal hearts in patients older than 30 years, especially under exercise testing, is reported to be associated with increased risk for sudden cardiac death.[2,3] PVCs and runs of nonsustained ventricular tachycardias in individuals with structural heart disease increases mortality risk.[4,5] Ablation is recommended[6] in patients who are at low risk for sudden cardiac death, have drug-resistant symptomatic predominantly monomorphic PVCs and/or nonsustained monomorphic ventricular tachycardia, or who are drug intolerant or refuse long-term drug therapy.

Preprocedural mapping of PVC origin is conventionally performed with the body surface 12-lead electrocardiogram (ECG). However, 12-lead ECG arrhythmia-origin algorithms have limitations and may negatively influence ablation outcome. For example, erroneous interpretation of the site or chamber of origin from the ECG (right or left ventricle) may result in unnecessary exploratory catheter mapping or failure to identify the treatable target. ECVUE (CardioInsight, Cleveland, OH), a three-dimensional, noninvasive, single-beat mapping system, offers a solution for preprocedure PVC characterization and localization with high accuracy, which has the potential to improve clinical outcome.

Conflict of Interest: T. Neumann has received speakers' honoraria from CardioInsight.
a Medical Clinic I, Department of Cardiology, Justus-Liebig University of Giessen, Klinikstrasse 33, Giessen 35392, Germany; b Department of Cardiology, Kerckhoff Heart and Thorax Center, Benekestr 2-8, Bad Nauheim 61231, Germany
* Corresponding author.
E-mail address: t.neumann@kerckhoff-klinik.de

NONINVASIVE PREMATURE VENTRICULAR COMPLEXES MAPPING: ECVUE TECHNOLOGY

The computational methods used in the reconstruction of ECVUE maps using multiple body surface electrodes have been described previously.[7] Briefly, a 252-electrode vest is applied to the patient's torso to record surface potentials. Following a noncontrast, low-dose thoracic computed tomography (CT) scan, the heart and vest electrodes are segmented. The electrode positions and three-dimensional epicardial biventricular geometry are used by the ECVUE system to reconstruct epicardial potentials and unipolar electrograms for each beat of interest.[8,9] The clinical PVC is processed by the ECVUE system to display a color-coded activation sequence of origin and propagation of the PVC beat. Several electrophysiologic characteristics are reviewed to confirm the diagnosis as follows: pattern or activation, where the chamber harboring the arrhythmia is the first to activate, whereas the passive chamber activates last (**Figs. 1** and **2**); and unipolar electrogram morphology at the earliest epicardial breakthrough, where presence of a large Q wave denotes epicardial origin and rS morphology denotes endocardial origin. A flow chart of the diagnostic algorithm for noninvasive mapping is in **Fig. 3**.

ABLATION ACCURACY AND SUCCESS

The feasibility and accuracy of PVC mapping using the ECVUE system has been previously reported.[10–12] Specifically, two studies compared accuracy of PVC mapping using ECVUE with the standard 12-lead body surface ECG.[10,11] In both studies, ECVUE was first used to localize the PVC origin to either the right or left chamber, and

second to sublocalize the origin within the ventricular chambers. Jamil-Copley and coworkers[10] conducted a prospective single-center study, which included 24 patients, most of whom had idiopathic PVCs emanating from the outflow tracts (**Fig. 4**). The ECVUE system was used to correctly identify the chamber and sublocalize the PVC origin in 96% of the cases. In contrast, using several established 12-lead body surface ECG algorithms,[13–15] accurate identification of chamber of PVC origin was achieved in only 50% to 88% of the cases and sublocalization within the right ventricular outflow tract (RVOT) in only 37% to 58%. Ground truth of PVC origin was established by an invasive electrophysiology study (EP).

More recently, Erkapic and colleagues[11] published a prospective randomized study including 42 patients (mostly idiopathic PVCs). Similar to Jamil-Copley and coworkers, Erkapic and colleagues found that established 12-lead ECG algorithms correctly identified the chamber harboring the PVC in only 76.2% of the cases compared with 95.2% with the ECVUE system. Moreover, accurate sublocalization of the ventricular arrhythmia within the chambers was significantly superior using ECVUE versus the standard 12-lead ECG (95.2% vs 38.1%, respectively; **Table 1**).

Accurate identification of PVC origin may be challenging even with the ECVUE system, especially for more septal locations. For example, in the studies of Jamil-Copley and coworkers[10] and Erkapic and colleagues,[11] ECVUE failed to correctly localize PVC origin in two patients (one patient in each study, respectively). Jamil-Copley and coworkers[10] reported ECVUE localization of the PVC origin at the inferoseptal RVOT, preprocedurally, but during the EP study, the PVC origin was identified in the left ventricular outflow tract

RVOT Sep

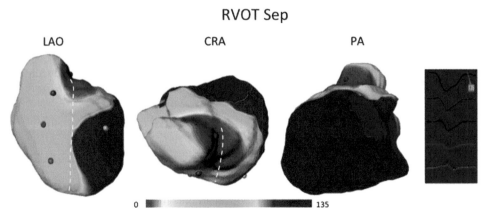

Fig. 1. PVC originating in the right ventricular outflow tract (RVOT). Activation maps of a PVC originating in the RVOT in left anterior oblique (LAO), cranial (CRA), and posterior-anterior (PA) views. Earliest activation is localized to the septal RVOT with a typical Q-wave morphology electrogram. Activation then rapidly spreads down the right ventricle, with the left ventricle activating last.

LVOT Sep

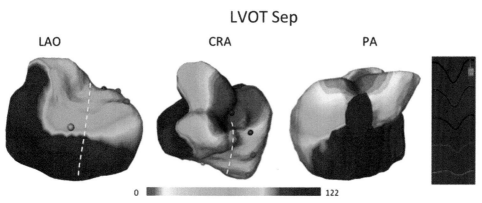

Fig. 2. PVC originating in the left ventricular outflow tract (LVOT). Activation maps of a PVC originating in the LVOT in LAO, CRA, and PA views. Earliest activation is localized to the septal RVOT with a typical Q-wave morphology electrogram. Activation then rapidly spreads down the left ventricle, with the right ventricle activating last.

(LVOT) between the right and noncoronary cusp. Similarly, Erkapic and colleagues[11] reported one incorrect ECVUE-guided PVC localization predicted to originate from the septal LVOT, but the arrhythmia was successfully mapped and ablated at the septal RVOT. Cakulev and colleagues[12] reported a series with 10 patients with PVCs, of whom eight PVC origins were correctly identified by ECVUE. In the two failed cases, suspected PVC origins were at the septal outflow tract region (one at RVOT posterosepal and one at LVOT), were never successfully ablated, and therefore the true PVC origin could not be verified.

CLINICAL IMPLICATIONS
Left Ventricular Outflow Tract/Right Ventricular Outflow Tract Premature Ventricular Complexes

PVCs that arise from the outflow tracts are not always straightforward to map and/or ablate. First,

the outflow tracts are in very close proximity to one another. Second, the myocardial network surrounding the ventricular outflow tracts is very complex. There are myocardial fibers connecting the outflow tracts with each other and fibers connecting the aortic cusps and the distal coronary sinus. Finally, the wide space between the ectopic origin and the endocardial breakout coupled with the fast propagation speeds in the outflow tracts can complicate accurate noninvasive and invasive mapping.

A natural question arises when interpreting the accuracy of PVC identification using established ECG algorithms: why is it so difficult to accurately predict PVC origin from the 12-lead ECG? The answer lies in the flawed fundamental assumption that all hearts and bodies are created equal (ie, the same sized heart lies in the same orientation within the same body habitus). Because people and their hearts come in all shapes and sizes, it is not at all surprising that even an experienced

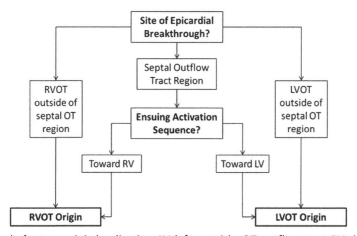

Fig. 3. ECVUE method of ectopy origin localization. LV, left ventricle; OT, outflow tract; RV, right ventricle. (*From* Jamil-Copley S, Bokan R, Kojodjojo P, et al. Noninvasive electrocardiographic mapping to guide ablation of outflow tract ventricular arrhythmias. Heart Rhythm 2014;11(4):587–94; with permission.)

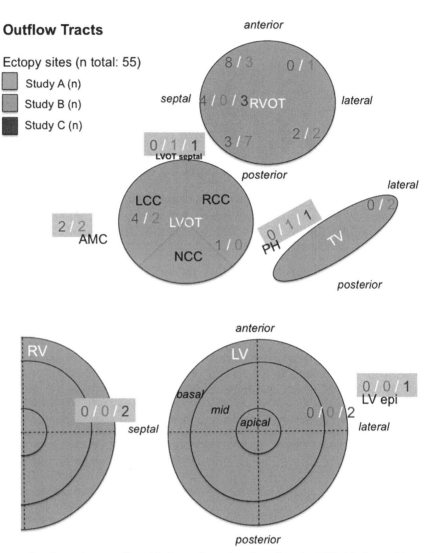

Fig. 4. PVC ectopy sites from three studies with three-dimensional noninvasive PVC ablation guidance (Study A[10]/ Study B[11]/Study C[12]). AMC, aortomitral continuity; epi, epicardial; LCC, left coronary cusp; LV, left ventricle; NCC, noncoronary cusp; PH, parahissian; RCC, right coronary cusp; RV, right ventricle; TV, tricuspid valve. (*Data from* Refs.[10–12])

Table 1			
Comparison of three-dimensional noninvasive guided PVC mapping with conventional (12-lead body surface ECG) mapping			
PVC Mapping Tool	**Patients (N)**	**Accuracy of Preprocedural PVC Chamber Localization (%)**	**Accuracy of Preprocedural PVC Sublocalization (%)**
12-lead ECG	24/21	50–88/76	37–58/38
ECVUE	24/21	96/95	96/95

Abbreviation: PVC, premature ventricular complex.

Data from Jamil-Copley S, Bokan R, Kojodjojo P, et al. Non-invasive electrocardiographic mapping to guide ablation of outflow tract ventricular arrhythmias. Heart Rhythm 2014;11:587–94; and Erkapic D, Greiss H, Pajitnev D, et al. Clinical impact of a novel three-dimensional electrocardiographic imaging for non-invasive mapping of ventricular arrhythmias-a prospective randomized trial. Europace 2014. [Epub ahead of print].

electrophysiologist can preprocedurally fail to accurately localize the origin of ventricular arrhythmia by using the standard 12-lead ECG algorithms. The advantage of the ECVUE's noninvasive three-dimensional mapping system is that PVCs are mapped in a single beat to a patient's individual heart torso geometry. Furthermore, by virtue of its dual-chamber geometry, ECVUE provides global activation patterns (ie, active chamber activates first while the passive chamber activates last) and electrogram (EGM) analyses as highlighted previously, which explain its superiority in identifying arrhythmia origin compared with the 12-lead ECG.

Comparison with Traditional Methods

Conventional invasive mapping and ablation of ventricular arrhythmias using sequential activation and pace mapping has known limitations.[16–18] It is reported that in approximately 20% of patients, pace mapping is unreliable in identifying the site of origin, possibly because of a deeper site of origin and preferential conduction via fibers connecting the focus to the endocardial surface.[17] The high mapping accuracy of the ECVUE system should be expected to positively influence ablation procedure by simplifying mapping, reducing ablation and procedural time, and as a result improving clinical outcome. Erkapic and colleagues[11] evaluated ECVUE's impact on procedural end points compared with conventional ablation by activation and pace mapping (without an invasive three-dimensional mapping system).

Indeed, ECVUE-guided ablation was proved to be more precise than conventional ablation. On average, the PVCs could be swiftly eliminated with the first radiofrequency (RF) application (followed by a safety application), whereas twice as many RF applications were required in the conventional group to achieve PVC elimination. Time to ablation was 35.3 minutes in the conventional group and 24.4 minutes in the ECVUE group (P = .035). Total procedure time (skin to skin) was also significant shorter in the ECVUE group (89 vs 78 minutes; P = .021). Furthermore, there were more PVC relapses during the requisite 30-minute waiting period in the conventional group (33.3%) versus the ECVUE group (14.3%), which further supports the increased accuracy of ECVUE-guided PVC identification (**Table 2**).

Accurate preprocedural localization of PVC origin may help avoid unnecessary and/or additional arterial or venous vascular access, which might be associated with lower complication risks. For example, Erkapic and colleagues[11] reported that incorrect localization of PVC origin in the 12-lead ECG group necessitated a modification of the vascular approach in 23.8% of the patients and only in 4.7% of the patients mapped with ECVUE. Of course, experienced operators were able to overcome the challenges associated with the conventional approach, and as a result, acute and chronic ablation success rates were similar in both groups.

Of note, the required CT scan for the ECVUE system increases overall radiation exposure in patients. Because of the current inability to visualize the ablation catheter on the ECVUE's CT geometry, operators must perform fluoroscopic-guided navigation or use an alternative invasive three-dimensional mapping system. But it is conceivable that using an invasive three-dimensional mapping system either only in the conventional group or in the ECVUE group could further reduce radiation exposure. Certainly, the ability to localize the PVC origin with only one beat is an advantage

Table 2
Comparison of conventional and ECVUE-guided ablation

	Conventional Ablation			ECVUE Guided Ablation			
	Median	Q1	Q3	Median	Q1	Q3	P Value
Total RF applications (N)	4	3	5	2	2	3	.005
Applications to first effect (N)	2	1	3	1	1	2	.023
Time to ablation (min)	35.3	22	47.8	24.4	11.3	35.3	.035
Skin-to-skin time (min)	89	73	114	78	64	100	.021
X-ray dose during EPS	0.39	0.16	0.78	0.36	0.14	0.69	.203
Total x-ray dose (mSV) (including CT scan)	0.39	0.16	0.78	3.21	2.93	3.70	.001

Abbreviations: EPS, electrophysiology study; Q, quartile.

Adapted from Erkapic D, Greiss H, Pajitnev D, et al. Clinical impact of a novel three-dimensional electrocardiographic imaging for non-invasive mapping of ventricular arrhythmias-a prospective randomized trial. Europace 2014. [Epub ahead of print].

not only over the conventional but also over invasive three-dimensional mapping systems, which use point-by-point activation mapping as guidance. Despite CT-related higher radiation exposure in the ECVUE group, in patients with symptomatic but low PVC burden, or in challenging redo cases, the ECVUE system has the potential to improve clinical outcome.

CHRONIC SUCCESS

Using preprocedural and postprocedural 24 hour holter monitoring, PVC burden showed significant reduction over a mean follow-up duration of 12 months in the study of Jamil-Copley and co-workers[10] and 3 months in the study of Erkapic and colleagues.[11]

Although the ability to accurately map the PVC to the site of origin is paramount, chronic ablation success depends on many factors, such as procedural RF settings. Of the reported 55 patients with PVC guided by the ECVUE system,[10–12] only six had symptomatic recurrences. The recurrences were likely caused by inappropriate RF power settings during ablation rather than incorrect three-dimensional noninvasive mapping. With appropriate power settings, the recurred PVCs were successfully reablated at the exact location previously identified by ECVUE. In the study of Cakulev and colleagues[12] both patients with failed ablation success exhibited transient suppression of the PVCs during ablation at the site of earliest activation. These sites were also predicted to be the origin of the PVC by ECVUE.

SUMMARY

ECVUE technology can accurately characterize and localize PVCs with performance superior to the body surface ECG, at the expense of increased patient radiation exposure because of the requisite CT scan. However, accurate preprocedure PVC localization plays an important role in planning the ablation strategy. For example, predicting the accurate chamber harboring the arrhythmia can help plan for appropriate left ventricle or right ventricle access, which can potentially reduce periprocedural risk (eg, embolic events). In addition, preprocedure mapping can help physicians better inform their patients about procedural time and risk. Because of its single-beat nature, ECVUE is also indispensable in mapping infrequent PVCs. Furthermore, current data demonstrate that accurate preprocedural PVC localization is responsible for increased ablation procedure efficacy attributable to fewer RF applications required to terminate PVCs, decreased time to first RF application, and decreased total procedure time. In conclusion, ECVUE noninvasively provides accurate PVC localization thereby enabling an effective treatment strategy.

REFERENCES

1. Hiss RG, Lamb LE. Electrocardiographic findings in 122,043 individuals. Circulation 1962;25:947–61.
2. Jouven X, Zureik M, Desnos M, et al. Long-term outcome in asymptomatic men with exercise-induced premature ventricular depolarizations. N Engl J Med 2000;343:826–33.
3. Frolkis JP, Pothier CE, Blackstone EH, et al. Frequent ventricular ectopy after exercise as a predictor of death. N Engl J Med 2003;348:781–90.
4. Ruberman W, Weinblatt E, Goldberg JD, et al. Ventricular premature complexes and sudden death after myocardial infarction. Circulation 1981;64:297–305.
5. Moss AJ, Hall WJ, Cannom DS, et al, for the Multicenter Automatic Defibrillator Implantation Trial Investigators. Improved survival with an implanted defibrillator in patients with coronary disease at high risk for ventricular arrhythmia. N Engl J Med 1996;335:1933–40.
6. Zipes DP, Camm AJ, Borggrefe M, et al. ACC/AHA/ESC 2006 guidelines for management of patients with ventricular arrhythmias and the prevention of sudden cardiac death. Circulation 2006;114(10):e385–484.
7. Oster HS, Taccardi B, Lux RL, et al. Noninvasive electrocardiographic imaging: reconstruction of epicardial potentials, electrograms, and isochrenes and localization of single and multiple electrocardiac events. Circulation 1997;96:1012–24.
8. Rudy Y, Oster HS. The electrocardiographic inverse problem. Crit Rev Biomed Eng 1992;20:25–45.
9. Rudy Y, Burnes JE. Noninvasive electrocardiographic imaging. Ann Noninvasive Electrocardiol 1999;4:340–59.
10. Jamil-Copley S, Bokan R, Kojodjojo P, et al. Noninvasive electrocardiographic mapping to guide ablation of outflow tract ventricular arrhythmias. Heart Rhythm 2014;11:587–94.
11. Erkapic D, Greiss H, Pajitnev D, et al. Clinical impact of a novel three-dimensional electrocardiographic imaging for non-invasive mapping of ventricular arrhythmias-a prospective randomized trial. Europace 2014. [Epub ahead of print].
12. Cakulev I, Sahadevan J, Arruda M, et al. Confirmation of novel noninvasive high-density electrocardiographic mapping with electrophysiology study. Circ Arrhythm Electrophysiol 2013;6:68–75.
13. Betensky BP, Park RE, Marchlinski FE, et al. The V2 transition ratio: a new electrocardiographic criterion for distinguishing left from right ventricular outflow tract tachycardia origin. J Am Coll Cardiol 2011;57:2255–62.
14. Zhang F, Chen M, Yang B, et al. Electrocardiographic algorithm to identify the optimal target

ablation site for idiopathic right ventricular outflow tract ventricular premature contraction. Europace 2009;11:1214–20.

15. Ito S, Tada H, Naito S, et al. Development and validation of an ECG algorithm for identifying the optimal ablation site for idiopathic ventricular outflow tract tachycardia. J Cardiovasc Electrophysiol 2003; 14:1280–6.

16. De Ponti R, Ho SY. Mapping of right ventricular outflow tract tachycardia/ectopies: activation mapping vs. pace mapping. Heart Rhythm 2008; 5:345–7.

17. Bogun F, Taj M, Ting M, et al. Spatial resolution of pace mapping of idiopathic ventricular tachycardia/ectopy originating in the right ventricular outflow tract. Heart Rhythm 2008;5:339–44.

18. Zhang F, Yang B, Chen H, et al. Noncontact mapping to guide ablation of right ventricular outflow tract arrhythmias. Heart Rhythm 2013; 12:1895–902.

Utility of Noninvasive Arrhythmia Mapping in Patients with Adult Congenital Heart Disease

Sabine Ernst, MD, FESC[a,b,*], Johan Saenen, MD[a],
Riikka Rydman, MD[a], Federico Gomez, MD[a],
Karine Roy, MD[a], Lilian Mantziari, MD[a],
Irina Suman-Horduna, MD[a]

KEYWORDS

- Congenital heart disease • Catheter ablation • Anatomy • Three-dimensional mapping
- Noninvasive • Outcomes

KEY POINTS

- Previous body surface mapping approaches lacked integration of the individual anatomy, and therefore have rarely been used in clinical practice in the last decade.
- A recently introduced noninvasive multielectrode electrocardiographic mapping system (ECVUE; CardioInsight Technologies Inc, Cleveland, OH, USA) combines 3-dimensional (3D) reconstruction of the cardiac anatomy from computed tomography scans with simultaneous recording of the cardiac activation from 252 surface electrocardiographic electrograms.
- The noninvasive nature of the 3D multielectrode mapping system helped to differentiate multiple targets in some patients or rare ectopy over a longer mapping time of several hours.
- Documentation of the location of the critical substrate allowed an informed choice regarding conventional versus remote-controlled navigation techniques, which in turn resulted in limited procedure time and radiation exposure.
- The 3D multielectrode mapping system helped avoid the unnecessary risk of an invasive procedure in patients with palpitations resulting from sinus tachycardia.

INTRODUCTION

Arrhythmia management in patients with adult congenital heart disease (ACHD) is a challenge on many levels, as tachycardic episodes may lead to hemodynamic impairment in otherwise compensated patients even if episodes are only transient.[1,2] Arrhythmias are in all the different types of congenital cohorts a marker for significant morbidity and mortality.[2–6] Owing to the underlying condition, challenges can present in various aspects such as the corrected anatomic situation after surgery, the inherent conduction properties of a potentially abnormally located or otherwise impaired conduction system, and the arrhythmia substrate itself in the form of fibrosis and/or surgically acquired scars.[7] This presentation may give rise to a multitude of arrhythmia

The authors have nothing to disclose.
[a] Department of Cardiology, Royal Brompton Hospital, Sydney Street, London SW3 6NP, UK; [b] NIHR Cardiovascular Biomedical Research Unit, Royal Brompton and Harefield Hospital, National Heart and Lung Institute, Imperial College London, Sydney Street, London SW3 6NP, UK
* Corresponding author. Royal Brompton and Harefield Hospital, National Heart and Lung Institute, Imperial College London, Sydney Street, London SW3 6NP, UK.
E-mail address: s.ernst@rbht.nhs.uk

Card Electrophysiol Clin 7 (2015) 117–123
http://dx.doi.org/10.1016/j.ccep.2014.11.007
1877-9182/15/$ – see front matter © 2015 Elsevier Inc. All rights reserved.

substrates, which can vary from infrequent atrial or ventricular ectopy to sustained reentrant tachycardias.[3,8–10] Some congenital conditions, such as Ebstein anomaly, have a high incidence of multiple accessory pathways, giving rise to atrioventricular (AV) reentrant tachycardia; this may include several accessory pathways or the normal conduction system, resulting in variable AV reentrant circuits, which can confuse the invasive electrophysiologist and increase the complexity of any catheter ablation procedure.[11,12] However, as ACHD patients are usually young and active members of society, any curative approach to their arrhythmias leads to a dramatic change in their clinical course such that catheter ablation is advocated in preference to lifelong antiarrhythmic medication by many interventional electrophysiologists. Recently several technical advances, including 3-dimensional (3D) image integration, 3D mapping, and remote magnetic navigation, have been introduced to facilitate curatively intended ablation procedures in this special patient cohort.[13–15] This review attempts to outline the role of a novel technology of simultaneous, noninvasive mapping in this patient cohort, and gives details of the authors' single-center experience.[16–18]

SIMULTANEOUS VERSUS SEQUENTIAL MAPPING

To allow successful catheter ablation, a detailed understanding of the arrhythmia and the exact localization of the critical substrate (eg, focal source of the arrhythmia or critical isthmus of a reentry) needs to be identified.[7,19] Although body surface electrocardiogram (ECG) mapping has been available for a long time, most invasive mapping systems have used a sequential recording approach, which requires a stable arrhythmia.[15,20] Any infrequent, irregular, or unstable arrhythmia is essentially "nonmappable" using a sequential approach, as the activation pattern is constantly changing. Moreover, infrequently occurring arrhythmias that are difficult to provoke under catheter laboratory conditions pose a challenge in the electrophysiology (EP) laboratory, as the physiologic conditions of the sympathetic drive might be diminished, especially if invasive procedures require sedation of the patient.

Body surface mapping approaches of the past lacked the integration of the individual anatomy, and therefore have been used rarely in clinical practice in the last decade. The recent introduction of the noninvasive multielectrode ECG mapping (ECM) system (ECVUE; CardioInsight Technologies Inc, Cleveland, OH, USA) has now

closed this gap.[17,18] It combines the 3D reconstruction of the cardiac anatomy from computed tomography (CT) scans with the simultaneous recording of the cardiac activation from 252 surface ECG electrograms. Using an inverse solution, virtual unipolar electrograms are reconstructed on the epicardial surface of either the atrial or ventricular chambers. This panoramic mapping system allows assessment of a global activation sequence from a single beat in a noninvasive fashion. Its use so far has been reported in patients with atrial or ventricular tachycardia, accessory pathway dependent tachycardia, and atrial fibrillation.

METHODS
Patient Population

Of a total cohort of 27 patients undergoing ECM at the authors' institution from November 2012 to May 2013, 14 had an underlying ACHD condition. **Table 1** gives an overview of the detailed conditions. Patients were recruited from the waiting list for invasive EP studies and gave consent for the noninvasive mapping study using the ECM in addition to the invasive EP procedure. In cases of rare

Table 1
Demographics of patients with adult congenital heart disease

No. of patients	14
Age (y)	32.8 (24.6–47.4)
Gender	9 F, 5 M
Underlying heart disease	1 D-TGA + arterial switch 2 CCTGA 1 AVSD 1 LSVC + mitral valve disease 1 DiGeorge syndrome 2 Coarctation of the aorta 2 Fontan 2 Ebstein 1 Double-chambered RV + VSD repair 1 ASD repair
Previous ablation	9 (6 AT/AF, 1 WPW, 2 VE)
Spontaneous ablation target	9
Provocation during EP study	12

Abbreviations: ASD, atrial septal defect; AT/AF, atrial tachycardia/atrial fibrillation; AVSD, atrioventricular septal defect; CCTGA, congenitally corrected transposition of the great arteries; D-TGA, dextro-transposition of the great arteries; EP, electrophysiology; LSVC, left superior vena cava; RV, right ventricle; VE, ventricular ectopy; VSD, ventricular septal defect; WPW, Wolff-Parkinson-White syndrome.

or transient arrhythmias, all antiarrhythmic drugs were discontinued for at least 3 times the elimination half-life, whereas patients with persistent arrhythmia were rate-controlled only. If present, oral anticoagulation was paused 1 day before the procedure.

Preacquired Computed Tomography Image Acquisition and 3-Dimensional Reconstruction

A thoracic, noncontrast CT scan (Somatom; Siemens, Forchheim, Germany) was acquired with the multielectrode vest attached to the patient, firstly to exactly locate the surface electrodes and secondly to reconstruct the 3D anatomy of the atrial or ventricular chambers. Landmarks including the atrioventricular valves, left anterior descending artery (LAD), and posterior descending artery (PDA) were added to facilitate orientation for the operator.

For each heart beat the ECM generated 1500 unipolar electrograms on the 3D epicardial reconstruction of the heart, giving rise to color-coded isopotential, voltage, and propagation maps. The maximal negative slope of the local electrograms determined the activation time, allowing the generation of isochronal and directional activation maps.

Arrhythmia Recording Using Noninvasive Electrocardiographic Mapping

In all cases, patients underwent a recording period on the ward to document their clinical arrhythmia outside the catheter laboratory. In case of rare or transient palpitations, several maneuvers were attempted to provoke arrhythmias, including bicycle exercise, vagal stimulation, and hyperventilation. If the patient remained noninducible, pharmacologic provocation was attempted with isoprenaline infusion and/or atropine injection.

Details of the Invasive Electrophysiology Study

Patients with inducible or spontaneously occurring arrhythmias were brought to the EP laboratory. Depending on the underlying heart disease, type of arrhythmia, and the necessity to exclude intracardiac thrombi by transesophageal echocardiography, the procedure was performed under local anesthetic, sedation, or general anesthesia as per institutional standards.

At the beginning of the EP study, conventional programmed stimulation was carried via diagnostic catheters to evaluate the basic electrical properties. In the case of sustained spontaneous or induced arrhythmia, appropriate conventional pacing maneuvers were performed to ascertain the critical isthmus, and all conventional

electrograms were recorded on a conventional recording system (Siemens AG, Forchheim, Germany) in parallel with the ECM recordings. If deemed necessary by the operator, the remote-controlled navigation system Niobe (Stereotaxis Inc, St Louis, MO, USA) was used in conjunction with the ECM system. Details of this system have been described previously[13,14] for patients with normal or congenital heart disease.

RESULTS

A total of 14 patients with ACHD (mean age 37.4 ± 18.3 years, 9 female) underwent noninvasive mapping using the ECM in preparation for their EP study. Diagnosis of ACHD ranged from left atrial isomerism to tricuspid atresia with right atrium, pulmonary artery Fontan operation, aortic coarctation, and arterial switch for dextro-transposition of the great arteries (see **Table 1**). Only 5 patients had no previous ablation attempt while the majority had failed at least 1 previous sequential EP study.

Noninvasive Multielectrode Mapping Outside the Catheter Laboratory

Half of the patients presented with ongoing or spontaneously occurring arrhythmia (**Fig. 1**), and 6 of the arrhythmias originated from the ventricular myocardium and 7 from the atrium, respectively. One patient demonstrated overt preexcitation of a posterolateral accessory pathway in the presence of Ebstein anomaly. In 5 patients, additional measures were taken to induce any arrhythmia; these included physiologic maneuvers (hand grip, Valsalva), physical activity (rapid pace walking, riding a stationary bicycle), or pharmacologic provocation with isoprenaline infusion or atropine bolus. One case with previously documented ventricular ectopics was found to be noninducible and was referred to the EP laboratory since a 12-lead ECG of the clinical ventricular ectopic morphology had been documented earlier, and 1 case was excluded from further study because no arrhythmias were observed at baseline and nothing other than sinus tachycardia could be induced by exercise or pharmacologic provocation. The accelerated sinus rhythm correlated well with the clinical symptoms of these patients, who had undergone several ablation procedures previously, such that no further invasive EP approach was pursued.

In Vivo Localization of the Ablation Target

As the ECM is not a navigation system in the classic sense, no depiction of the ablation catheter

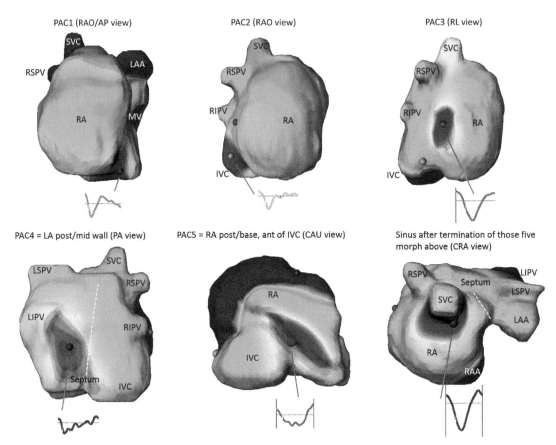

Fig. 1. Example of a 29-year-old female patient with tricuspid and pulmonary atresia. Five different premature atrial contractions (PACs) were mapped and successfully ablated. Red shows earliest breakthrough; blue/purple shows late activation. AP, anteroposterior; CAU, caudal; CRA, cranial; IVC, inferior vena cava; LA, left anterior; LAA, left atrial appendage; LIPV, left inferior pulmonary vein; LSPV, left superior pulmonary vein; MV, mitral valve; PA, posteroanterior; RA, right atrium; RAA, right atrial appendage; RAO, right anterior oblique; RIPV, right inferior pulmonary vein; RL, right lateral; RSPV, right superior pulmonary vein; SVC, superior vena cava.

localization is available. Navigation toward the ablation target is helped by iterative spike or pace-mapping techniques. In the first case, pacing is required via the mapping catheter and encompasses the epicardial mapping of the pacing spike with the ECVUE.[21] As only the site of earliest activation is informative for revealing the position of the mapping catheter, only the pacing spike is used for this approach. Moreover, pace match was visually evaluated to compare the isopotential map of the paced beat with that of a spontaneous beat (**Fig. 2**). The substrate of interest was further confirmed by classic entrainment and pace-mapping maneuvers. The ECM guided the positioning of the mapping catheter while probing for positive entrainment and perfect pace match, and showed great precision as warming up was observed on radiofrequency (RF) application in many of the designated target areas.

Combination of Magnetic Navigation and ECVUE

In many patients with ACHD, the use of the magnetic navigation system has been advantageous in overcoming access problems, as reported recently.[14,22] In these studies, the authors elected to use the remote magnetic navigation combined with ECVUE-guided mapping in 4 patients. To the best of their knowledge, this is the first report of the combination of remote magnetic navigation with the ECM platform. The advantages to this patient cohort are evident, as the ECM allows fast arrhythmia mapping regardless of accessibility or anatomic complexity together with remote navigation, further reducing radiation exposure and enhancing access to less favorable anatomy such as corrected congenital heart disease. In the authors' experience, the magnetic field does not

Potential Maps (RAO view)

1. Bedside 3 beats PVC mapped as same morph simultaneously having epicardial breakthrough at the RV basal and ant side, septally. Presented area is close to the Sinus breakout level. Suspecting the RV septum close to the conducting system.

2. Invasively, PM at the para-HIS location (yellow marker on RAO/LAO projection). Map shows similar simultaneously epicardial breakthrough at the RV basal and ant side, however, not presenting the same inf/sep RV activation/propagation.

3. Invasively, PM at the position of white marker (ref. RAO/LAO projection). Map shows similar simultaneously epicardial breakthrough at the RV basal and ant side, however, not presenting the same inf/sep RV activation/propagation.

4. Best PM just 1cm below the HIS (light blue marker in RAO/LAO). RF on to see the warming up and first time clinical ectopy (mapped to confirm the same morphology)

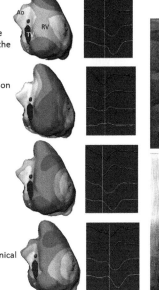
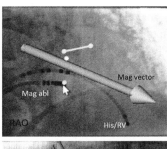
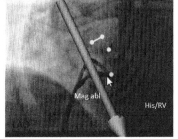

Fig. 2. Spontaneous ventricular ectopic and iterative pace map to locate the focal origin using the ECM in combination with remote magnetic navigation. Ao, aorta; HIS, His recording electrodes; LAO, left anterior oblique; Mag, magnetic mapping and ablation catheter; PA, pulmonary artery; PM, pace map; PVC, premature ventricular contraction; RAO, right anterior oblique; RF, radiofrequency; RV, right ventricle/ventricular; TV, tricuspid valve.

cause noise after the magnetic vector has moved, or interference that precludes the use of the ECVUE platform.

Outcome of ECVUE-Guided Ablation in Patients with Adult Congenital Heart Disease

All but 1 patient finally were studied invasively, with only 5 patients under general anesthesia and the remainder under assisted sedation by a dedicated cardiac anesthetic team. Procedure duration amounted to a median 188 minutes (interquartile range 164–237 minutes). Median fluoroscopy duration was 14.7 minutes (interquartile range 11.6–21.1 minutes) with a median of 20 RF applications. In 9 patients multiple arrhythmias were the target, which was greatly facilitated by the simultaneous mapping system. At follow-up (median of 18 months), 9 of 14 patients were in sinus rhythm while 3 experienced further arrhythmias despite antiarrhythmic medication. Of the 2 patients who were noninducible (1 on the ward without an invasive EP study and 1 who remained noninducible despite invasive EP study), both reported further nonsustained palpitations.

DISCUSSION

The recently introduced 3D noninvasive ECM system has the potential to overcome some of the limitations that hamper current ablation procedures.[16–18] The system overcomes several limitations that are currently not addressed by sequential mapping systems. First, this platform allows prolonged bedside monitoring in a noninvasive fashion and in more physiologic conditions. It allows one to challenge the patient with "common life situations" such as exercise or interaction with staff and relatives. This approach is extremely helpful especially during transient events, when patients can identify their typical symptoms. In the absence of any inducible or targetable arrhythmia, ECM was able to document, for example, sinus tachycardia (which for some patients is very symptomatic), thereby negating the need for further invasive procedures.

Furthermore, as the system requires a single beat to create a complete activation map, the ECM platform allows mapping of multiple arrhythmias in a limited time frame. It therefore is especially suitable for patients with congenital heart disease who often present with multiple arrhythmias. Hence in most patients the nature, number, and localization (ie, right- vs left-sided chamber, endo- vs epicardial surface) of the arrhythmia targets was identified even before the patient entered the EP laboratory, which is advantageous to procedural planning and execution, and prevents unnecessary risk of complications.

Despite the complexity of the underlying disease and the multitude of arrhythmias that were present in these patients, an overall acute success of 75% in a congenital heart disease cohort is impressive (excluding the noninducible patients from the analysis). Similar success rates were obtained for both atrial and ventricular arrhythmias. In the authors' hands, the combination with remote magnetic navigation is feasible and did not interfere with the operation of the ECM platform. In fact, it provided a further opportunity to reduce radiation exposure and allowed the operator to position the catheter in a stabilized fashion without risking dislodgment during the ECM analysis.

LIMITATIONS

The number of patients included in this study is modest; however, complex cases with extensive ACHD and multiple arrhythmias have been addressed here, making this novel technology at least an additional option to be considered in this challenging patient cohort. Better 3D reconstruction algorithms, especially for complex surgically corrected patients, are needed to allow better "road-map" guidance during the invasive part of the study.

SUMMARY

This article reports on the use of the ECM system for patients with ACHD for the treatment of both atrial and ventricular arrhythmias. In particular, the noninvasive nature of the 3D mapping process on the ward helped to differentiate multiple targets in some patients, or rare ectopy over a longer mapping time of several hours. Documentation of the location of the critical substrate then allowed an informed choice on conventional versus remote-controlled navigation techniques, which in turn resulted in limited procedure time and radiation exposure. This approach helped avoid the unnecessary risk of an invasive procedure in patients with palpitations caused by sinus tachycardia.

ACKNOWLEDGMENTS

The authors are indebted to Cheng Yao, PhD, who expertly supported the noninvasive and invasive part of these studies, as well as the preparation of the figures.

REFERENCES

1. Baumgartner H, Bonhoeffer P, De Groot NM, et al, Task Force on the Management of Grown-up Congenital Heart Disease of the European Society of Cardiology (ESC), Association for European Paediatric Cardiology (AEPC), ESC Committee for Practice Guidelines (CPG). ESC guidelines for the management of grown-up congenital heart disease (new version 2010). Eur Heart J 2010;31:2915–57.

2. Bernier M, Marelli AJ, Pilote L, et al. Atrial arrhythmias in adult patients with right- versus left-sided congenital heart disease anomalies. Am J Cardiol 2010;106:547–51.

3. Walsh EP. Interventional electrophysiology in patients with congenital heart disease. Circulation 2007;115:3224–34.

4. Gewillig M, Cullen S, Mertens B, et al. Risk factors for arrhythmia and death after mustard operation for simple transposition of the great arteries. Circulation 1991;84:III187–92.

5. Gatzoulis MA. Adult congenital heart disease: education, education, education. Nat Clin Pract Cardiovasc Med 2006;3:2–3.

6. Yap SC, Harris L. Sudden cardiac death in adults with congenital heart disease. Expert Rev Cardiovasc Ther 2009;7:1605–20.

7. Sherwin ED, Triedman JK, Walsh EP. Update on interventional electrophysiology in congenital heart disease: evolving solutions for complex hearts. Circ Arrhythm Electrophysiol 2013;6:1032–40.

8. Yap SC, Harris L, Silversides CK, et al. Outcome of intra-atrial re-entrant tachycardia catheter ablation in adults with congenital heart disease: negative impact of age and complex atrial surgery. J Am Coll Cardiol 2010;56:1589–96.

9. Morwood JG, Triedman JK, Berul CI, et al. Radiofrequency catheter ablation of ventricular tachycardia in children and young adults with congenital heart disease. Heart Rhythm 2004;1:301–8.

10. Triedman JK, Alexander ME, Love BA, et al. Influence of patient factors and ablative technologies on outcomes of radiofrequency ablation of intra-atrial re-entrant tachycardia in patients with congenital heart disease. J Am Coll Cardiol 2002;39:1827–35.

11. Legius B, Van De Bruaene A, Van Deyk K, et al. Behavior of Ebstein's anomaly: single-center experience and midterm follow-up. Cardiology 2010;117:90–5.

12. Roten L, Lukac P, DE Groot N, et al. Catheter ablation of arrhythmias in Ebstein's anomaly: a multi-center study. J Cardiovasc Electrophysiol 2011;22:1391–6.

13. Ueda A, Suman-Horduna I, Mantziari L, et al. Contemporary outcomes of supraventricular tachycardia ablation in congenital heart disease: a single-center experience in 116 patients. Circ Arrhythm Electrophysiol 2013;6:606–13.

14. Ernst S, Babu-Narayan SV, Keegan J, et al. Remote-controlled magnetic navigation and ablation with 3D image integration as an alternative approach in patients with intra-atrial baffle anatomy. Circ Arrhythm Electrophysiol 2012;5:131–9.

15. Triedman JK, DeLucca JM, Alexander ME, et al. Prospective trial of electroanatomically guided, irrigated catheter ablation of atrial tachycardia in patients with congenital heart disease. Heart Rhythm 2005;2: 700–5.
16. Ramanathan C, Jia P, Ghanem R, et al. Noninvasive electrocardiographic imaging (ECGI): application of the generalized minimal residual (GMRES) method. Ann Biomed Eng 2003;31:981–94.
17. Shah AJ, Hocini M, Xhaet O, et al. Validation of novel 3-dimensional electrocardiographic mapping of atrial tachycardias by invasive mapping and ablation: a multicenter study. J Am Coll Cardiol 2013;62:889–97.
18. Cuculich PS, Wang Y, Lindsay BD, et al. Noninvasive characterization of epicardial activation in humans with diverse atrial fibrillation patterns. Circulation 2010;122:1364–72.
19. Triedman JK, Alexander ME, Berul CI, et al. Electroanatomic mapping of entrained and exit zones in patients with repaired congenital heart disease and intra-atrial reentrant tachycardia. Circulation 2001;103:2060–5.
20. Rudy Y, Taccardi B. Noninvasive imaging and catheter imaging of potentials, electrograms, and isochrones on the ventricular surfaces. J Electrocardiol 1998;30(Suppl):19–23.
21. Jamil-Copley S, Bokan R, Kojodjojo P, et al. Noninvasive electrocardiographic mapping to guide ablation of outflow tract ventricular arrhythmias. Heart Rhythm 2014;11:587–94.
22. Ernst S, Ouyang F, Linder C, et al. Initial experience with remote catheter ablation using a novel magnetic navigation system: magnetic remote catheter ablation. Circulation 2004;109:1472–5.

Noninvasive Mapping of Electrical Dyssynchrony in Heart Failure and Cardiac Resynchronization Therapy

Niraj Varma, MD, PhD, FRCP[a],*, Sylvain Ploux, MD, PhD[b],
Philippe Ritter, MD[b], Bruce Wilkoff, MD[a],
Romain Eschalier, MD, PhD[b], Pierre Bordachar, MD, PhD[b]

KEYWORDS

- Electrocardiographic imaging ● LBBB ● Heart failure ● CRT ● LV activation mapping ● RV pacing

KEY POINTS

- Causes for diverse effects of cardiac resynchronization therapy (CRT) are poorly understood.
- Because CRT is an electrical treatment of an electrical disorder, attention to the electrical substrate and its interaction with pacing may be important. In support, electrocardiogram (ECG) features (morphology and duration) affect CRT outcomes; however, the surface ECG reports rudimentary electrical data.
- Noninvasive electrocardiographic imaging provides high-resolution, single-beat ventricular mapping, which reveals significant heterogeneity of left ventricle (LV) activation in patients with heart failure with wide QRS duration (≥120 milliseconds), coupled to unpredictable LV activation in response to biventricular pacing. Complex electrophysiologic barriers sometimes impede wave front propagation, and are not always related to scar. Several of these complex electrical characteristics, not decipherable from the 12-lead ECG, are linked to CRT effect.
- CRT response may be improved by candidate selection and LV lead placement directed by electrical evaluation on an individual basis.

INTRODUCTION

Cardiac resynchronization therapy (CRT) improves survival in patients with heart failure showing prolonged QRS duration.[1] The rationale underlying this therapy is that a prolonged QRS duration indicates late left ventricle (LV) activation, leading to intra-LV (septal vs lateral wall) and interventricular (LV vs right ventricle [RV]) dyssynchrony, to trigger adverse molecular remodeling and compromise mechanical function. Biventricular pacing is used to electrically resynchronize the ventricles. However, the persistence of a ~30% incidence of nonresponse over a decade of CRT practice, despite many attempts to ameliorate this condition by using measures of mechanical assessment,[2] indicates that current selection methods and/or pacing techniques are imperfect.

Limitations of the Surface QRS from the 12-Lead Electrocardiogram

Although CRT is intended to improve mechanical function, it is essentially an electrical therapy

Disclosures: This work was partly supported by grant R01-HL-49054 from the National Heart, Lung, and Blood Institute of the National Institutes of Health, USA.
[a] Cleveland Clinic, 9500 Euclid Avenue, Cleveland, OH 44195, USA; [b] CHU Bordeaux, Liryc Institute Bordeaux, Université de Bordeaux, France
* Corresponding author. J2-2, HVI, Cardiac Electrophysiology, Cleveland Clinic, 9500 Euclid Avenue, Cleveland, OH 44195.
E-mail address: varman@ccf.org

directed toward an electrical disorder, with transduced hemodynamic effects. Thus, candidate selection still depends on the electrical measure of the QRS. This electrical measure has recently been refined. For instance, QRS duration is only a reflection on the body surface of the total duration of ventricular activation and not a reliable marker of LV activation. Logically, patients with only RV delay should not benefit, and this has been confirmed in recent trials. Patients with right bundle branch block (RBBB) did not benefit from CRT.[3] In contrast, those candidates with left bundle branch block (LBBB) and wider QRS (eg, >150 milliseconds) have greater LV activation delay (eg, >95 milliseconds), and should derive greater benefit from CRT.[4,5] This finding too was supported by trial data and incorporated into guidelines. Nevertheless, not all patients with LBBB and QRS greater than 150 milliseconds gain benefit, and uncertainty remains about CRT outcomes for patients with QRS duration between 120 and 150 milliseconds.[6] Thus, current criteria, although showing the importance of electrical parameters, remain insufficient, which may reflect the limitations of the surface QRS.

Noninvasive Biventricular Electrical Mapping

More precise characterization of electrical substrate and also of responses to pacing may be fundamental to understanding CRT effect. This characterization is integral to candidate selection, deployment of pacing electrodes, and programming, but represents a line of inquiry that has been underexamined. It has been explored recently with a validated technique for detailed noninvasive electrical mapping of ventricular activation (electrocardiographic imaging [ECGI[7]]). This technique has shown that both substrate and its reaction to pacing are highly patient specific, and a one-size–fits-all strategy applied to any group of potential CRT candidates yields diverse responses.

Electrocardiographic Imaging Methodology

ECGI provides noninvasive high-resolution electrical mapping of cardiac excitation on the epicardial surface. ECGI images epicardial potentials, electrograms, isochrones (activation sequences), and repolarization patterns from body-surface electrocardiographic measurements. The system has been validated extensively both experimentally and in humans by comparison with direct epicardial mapping during open-heart surgery and with catheter mapping. Reconstruction accuracy superior to 10 mm was consistently obtained in humans. ECGI may therefore be used as a noninvasive

imaging modality for evaluation of human ventricle cardiac activation under differing conditions. The methodology has been detailed previously.[7,8] ECGI acquires more than 200 channels of body-surface electrocardiograms (ECGs) using a multielectrode vest. Epicardial geometry and body-surface electrode positions are registered simultaneously by a thoracic computed tomography scan. The body-surface potential data and the geometry data are processed with algorithms developed to compute epicardial potentials over the entire epicardium, from which epicardial electrograms (typically 600 over the heart surface), isochrones, and repolarization patterns are constructed. All images are obtained during a single beat.

REDEFINING LEFT BUNDLE BRANCH BLOCK

QRS duration is tightly correlated with time to terminal LV activation in LBBB (but not in RBBB).[4] This interval (qLV) sums 2 separate components: transseptal activation time and LV free wall activation time. Patients with LBBB by definition have delayed LV activation, conceived as a delay in transseptal transit of ventricular activation initiated by the right bundle branch (RBB; intact RBB conduction is responsible for rapid initial forces) (Fig. 1). Electrocardiographic mapping investigations of LBBB based on criteria used in the main CRT trials (QRS duration more than 120 milliseconds; RsR' in lead V_6 and rS/QS in V_1 or V_2) showed large variability in LV delay. Although RBB conduction and RV activation were well preserved, transseptal conduction could be rapid or delayed, and the following LV activation patterns were remarkably variable.[9,10]

In contrast, when applying more strict ECG criteria to the definition of the LBBB (eg, broad notched or slurred R wave in leads I, aVL, V_5, and V_6; and R peak time >60 milliseconds in leads V_5 and V_6), detailed electrical mapping revealed a fairly homogeneous pattern of the ventricular activation (Fig. 2). This pattern was characterized by a unique RV breakthrough, presence of lines of conduction delay, a laterobasal latest activated area, and a consistent delay of more than 50 milliseconds between the mean activation time of the two ventricles. These features have been shown to be associated with an increased probability of response. ECGI may therefore help to refine the LBBB definition and thus the selection reliability for CRT.

Features of Left Ventricle Activation Influencing Candidate Selection

In one study, a U-shaped LV activation pattern (ie, forced by an anterior conduction barrier), which

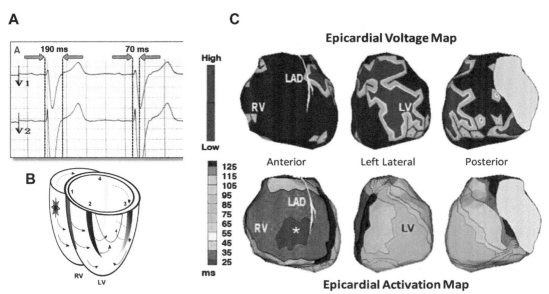

Fig. 1. Typical electrical activation during LBBB diagnosed by strict surface ECG criteria. (*A*) The 70-millisecond rS duration in V1/V2 indicates rapid initial myocardial activation via intact right bundle branch despite LBBB. (*B*) The right ventricular breakthrough is anterior or lateral. There is no left ventricular breakthrough. The LV is activated by anterior and posterior wave fronts originating from the RV. Between 1 and 4 lines of slow conduction with a base-to-apex orientation markedly delay the left ventricular epicardial activation and confine the end of activation to the lateral base. The star indicates right ventricular breakthrough; arrows indicate the direction of the activation wave fronts. 1, anteroseptal line; 2, anterolateral line; 3, posterolateral line; 4, one-quarter posteroseptal line. (*C*) ECGI maps: epicardial surfaces of both ventricles are displayed in 3 views. Anterior depicts the right ventricular free wall. The left anterior descending artery (LAD) is marked. (*Top panels*) Normal RV epicardial voltage (blue, anteriorly) contrasts with extensive left ventricular disease (*red zones*). (*Bottom*) RV breakthrough (*asterisk*) occurs laterally within 25 milliseconds. After this, RV activation is even, radial, and rapid (widely spaced isochrones), and completes within 45 milliseconds. The LV is then depolarized. Black areas indicate line/region of conduction block. The anteroseptal boundary marks the septal delay, following which LV is activated. (*From [A, C]* Varma N, Jia P, Ramanathan C, et al. RV electrical activation in heart failure during right, left, and biventricular pacing. JACC Cardiovasc Imaging 2010;3(6):570, with permission; and [*B*] Ploux S, Lumens J, Whinnett Z, et al. Noninvasive electrocardiographic mapping to improve patient selection for cardiac resynchronization therapy: Beyond QRS duration and left bundle-branch block morphology. J Am Coll Cardiol 2013;61(24):2438, with permission.)

has also been reported based on endocardial mapping, correlated with superior CRT effect.[9] A large area of latest activation (ie, terminal isochronal activity; eg, dark blue area in **Fig. 2**D) was correlated with greater increases in contractility in response to LV pacing.[11] Activation sequences perturbing papillary muscle function may cause mitral regurgitation and be rectified by LV preexcitation pacing.[12] These features are readily characterized by ECGI.

Measure of Electrical Dyssynchrony

Many time-dependent electrical dyssynchrony parameters have been examined. Esyn (the difference between the mean activation times of both ventricles) and ED (the standard deviation of the LV activation times) have been shown to be reduced by biventricular pacing.[13,14] The best tested metric to date has been the ventricular electrical uncoupling (VEU), defined as the difference

between the mean LV and RV activation times during spontaneous rhythm (in milliseconds). A positive value reflects LV uncoupling (from the RV), whereas a negative value reflects RV uncoupling (from the LV). A VEU value greater than 50 milliseconds was associated with a 42-fold increase in the likelihood of being a responder (*P*<.001), and behaved as a more powerful predictor than measurements made on the 12-lead ECG.[15] This finding suggests that electrical uncoupling of the LV from the RV is a fundamental component of the electrical substrate, which is amenable to treatment with CRT.

LEFT VENTRICULAR PACING

In addition to patient selection, using an optimal LV site for pacing may be a critical factor to CRT response. In current practice, LV lead placement at a site with good paced capture thresholds is

128

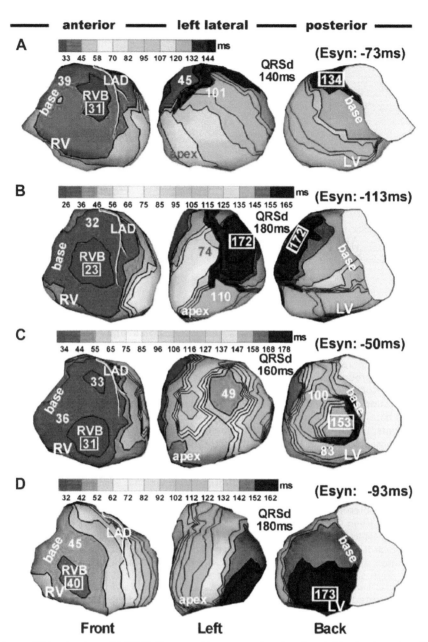

Fig. 2. Variations of LV activation with LBBB diagnosed by conventional surface ECG criteria. Epicardial isochrone maps of both ventricles for 4 representative patients are displayed in 3 views: anterior, left lateral, and posterior. There is overlap between adjacent views. LAD coronary artery is shown. Thick black markings indicate line/region of conduction block. Epicardial activation first occurred in the RV free wall. Following this, there was a rapid radial pattern of spread of activation from the zone of breakthrough (similarly to normal hearts[7,29]). RV activation is followed by delayed LV activation, indicating LBBB. Several different LV activation patterns are depicted. LV activation sometimes occurred from multiple directions (*C*). In others, activation spread from the anterior LV directly to the inferior LV (*D*), or the reverse (*A, B*). Wave front propagation was sometimes influenced by lines/regions of conduction block or slowed conduction. (Some lines remained unchanged with subsequent pacing, indicating fixed boundaries possibly generated by scar or otherwise nonconducting myocardial tissue. On other occasions, lines/regions of block shifted to other locations, disappeared, or emerged later during pacing maneuvers, suggesting a functional mechanism that did not correlate with scar distribution.) Lines of block could be multiple, generating complex conduction barriers. LV activation usually ended posterolaterally. These variations are not reflected in LBBB QRS configurations on surface electrocardiography. Electrical Synchrony Index (Esyn or VEU), corresponds with the mean activation time difference between lateral RV and LV free walls (ie, indexes interventricular resynchronization directly from measurements on the heart). Interventricular synchrony is indicated when Esyn equals zero, RV preexcitation by a negative Esyn, and LV preexcitation by positive Esyn value. QRSd, QRS duration; RVB, RV breakthrough. (*From* Jia P, Ramanathan C, Ghanem RN, et al. Electrocardiographic imaging of cardiac resynchronization therapy in heart failure: observation of variable electrophysiologic responses. Heart Rhythm 2006;3(3):300; with permission.)

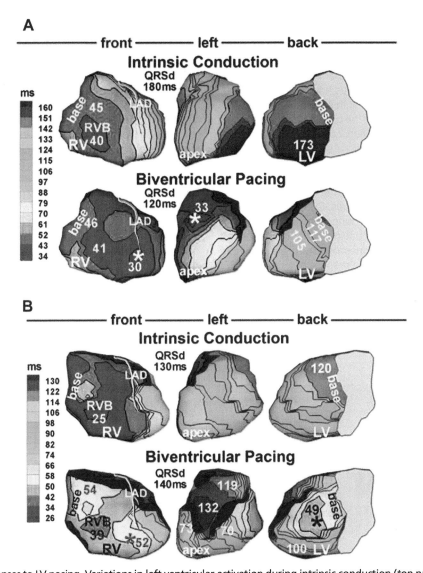

Fig. 3. Responses to LV pacing. Variations in left ventricular activation during intrinsic conduction (*top panels*) and biventricular pacing (*bottom panels*) are shown in 2 patients: a responder (*A*) and nonresponder (*B*) to CRT. Ventricular epicardial isochrone activation maps are shown using ECGI. Epicardial surfaces of both ventricles are displayed in 3 views: front, left, and back. There is overlap between adjacent views. The LAD coronary artery is shown. Thick black markings indicate line/region of conduction block. Pacing sites are marked by asterisks. (*Top panels*) Intrinsic conduction during LBBB. In both patients, ventricular activation of the RV begins with RVB and is followed by delayed (but even) LV activation, indicating LBBB. LV activation patterns differed. (*A*) There is even isochronal spread across the anterior LV surface (*left lateral view*), which then directs inferiorly. Terminal activation is at the inferolateral LV base (*back view*) 173 milliseconds after QRS onset. (*B*) The propagating wave front from the RV pivots around an anterior line of block so that LV activation commences from the apex and terminates at the anterolateral LV base 120 milliseconds after QRS onset. (*Bottom panels*) Responses to biventricular pacing (CRT). (*A*) In this CRT responder, activation spread rapidly from the anterior LV pacing site and ended at the basal LV after 117 milliseconds. A short line of block emerges in the anterolateral LV that was absent during intrinsic conduction. This line of block did not preclude response to CRT because posterolateral LV activation occurred rapidly and confluently, indicated by widely spaced isochrones across the bulk of the LV. Terminal posterolateral LV activation occurred at 117 milliseconds (shorter than during intrinsic conduction), so the intended effect of preexcitation LV pacing was achieved. (*B*) During biventricular pacing, lines of block emerge both anteriorly and across the anterolateral LV wall in this nonresponder to CRT. These lines were not evident during intrinsic conduction, indicating a functional mechanism. They prevent confluent LV activation, which occurs slowly, indicated by crowded isochrones, and are different from rapid even spread of LV activation during intrinsic conduction. Terminal LV activation occurs anteroseptally 132 milliseconds after pacing stimulus. Thus, posterolateral LV pacing slowed and dispersed the paced wave front in the lateral LV wall, in contrast with intrinsic conduction when conduction was rapid in the same area. QRS duration was prolonged. (*From* Varma N. Cardiac resynchronization therapy and the electrical substrate in heart failure: what does the QRS conceal? Heart Rhythm 2009;6:1059–62; with permission. *Adapted from* Jia P, Ramanathan C, Ghanem RN, et al. Electrocardiographic imaging of cardiac resynchronization therapy in heart failure: observation of variable electrophysiologic responses. Heart Rhythm 2006;3(3):302–303.)

regarded as effective lead placement. This approach assumes that LV pacing from an area of terminal LV activation causes homogeneous global LV activation (**Fig. 3**A), but this has been little characterized. For example, the presence of LV disease may modulate propagation. Most obviously, pacing into posterolateral transmural scar may negate CRT effect.[16,17] Avoidance improves outcome. However, ECGI studies have disclosed that LV activation even in the absence of scar may be unpredictable among, and within, individuals. Conduction barriers existing in nonscar areas during intrinsic conduction may be consolidated by pacing, or, more frequently, dissolved. Note that zones of conduction slowing and block may develop in response to pacing.

Fig. 3B shows poor LV activation in response to an anatomically ideal LV stimulation site. Although the posterolateral location has been advocated as most desirable, this has not been examined in detail. Such impediments to LV wave front propagation correlate with poorer hemodynamic response to pacing compared with when global activation was rapid[18] (ECGI may immediately reveal these effects, presaging lack of structural remodeling, irrespective of clinical symptoms[19]). Hemodynamics improved when these slow conduction areas were avoided and paced wave fronts were permitted to emerge and recruit adequate tissue mass.

In addition to these variations noted among individuals, slight changes in a single individual can dramatically affect LV activation patterns.

Striking changes in LV activation occurred without large electrode positional changes in any individual. For example, in **Fig. 4**, D1 and M2 poles were both sited posterolaterally in a

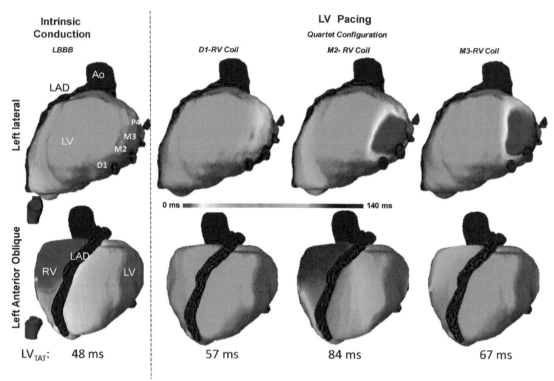

Fig. 4. Intraindividual variations in LV paced effects. The LV lead was a quadripolar electrode with ring electrodes at 20 mm (M2), 30 mm (M3), and 47 mm (P4) from the tip electrode (D1). LV pacing configurations using 3 separate LV poles (each to RV coil) are shown. These configurations have different effects, with conduction slowing in regions previously well activated during intrinsic conduction, indicating some functional properties of tissue. For example, D1-RV coil preexcites the posterior LV, after which LV activation is rapid. The anteroapical LV is activated in 57 milliseconds (note that RV apical activation follows without transseptal delay). In contrast, a slight shift (20 mm) in dipole from M2-RV coil changes the activation pattern significantly. The area of preexcitation is displaced anteriorly (*red area*), followed by fast lateral wall activation. However, propagation then encounters a zone of slow conduction anteroapically, indicated by crowded isochrones (color transition to *dark blue* isochrones across a short distance). These differences are reflected in more prolonged LV activation measures compared with D1-RV coil (LV$_{TAT}$ (LV total activation time), 84 vs 57 milliseconds; increased 47%). The M3-RV coil had intermediate effects. (*From* Varma N. Variegated left ventricular electrical activation in response to a novel quadripolar electrode: visualization by non-invasive electrocardiographic imaging. J Electrocardiol 2014;47(1):68; with permission.)

terminally activated region of the LV. Each would be considered an optimal lead site according to positional criteria, but reaction to pacing was very different. Because LV propagation patterns can be significantly altered by choice of pacing vector in any individual, LV depolarization in response to pacing is not necessarily constrained by the underlying intrinsic conduction disorder and/or cardiac disorder. These observations may explain why LV contractility (LV dp/dtmax) varied up to 2-fold between best-paced and worst-paced site (conducted without electrical mapping) and challenge an implant strategy simply targeting a late activated area (stimulation of which did not always yield maximum contractility improvement).[20,21] In view of these major interindividual and intraindividual variations in response to LV pacing, the pattern most likely to deliver the best long-term effect demands elucidation, and may direct an optimal implant strategy based on an individualized assessment of paced effect.

OUTSTANDING QUESTIONS IN CARDIAC RESYNCHRONIZATION THERAPY
Role of the Right Ventricular Pacing Electrode

Right ventricular pacing (either alone or in conjunction with simultaneous biventricular pacing) in patients with heart failure with LBBB significantly altered RV (and LV) activation compared with intrinsic conduction via the RBB,[10,22] delaying RV activation and perturbing natural centrifugal spread of activation (see **Fig. 3**B; **Fig. 5**). This effect may be avoided by LV pacing alone with critically timed atrioventricular (AV) delays resulting in fusion of the propagated paced wave front with intrinsic conduction via an intact right bundle. This CRT mode may avoid RV hemodynamic deficit associated with simultaneous biventricular pacing.[23] Pacing algorithms incorporating this feature may have long-term advantages.[24] However, ECGI revealed that, in some instances, the RV pacing electrode removed transseptal barriers

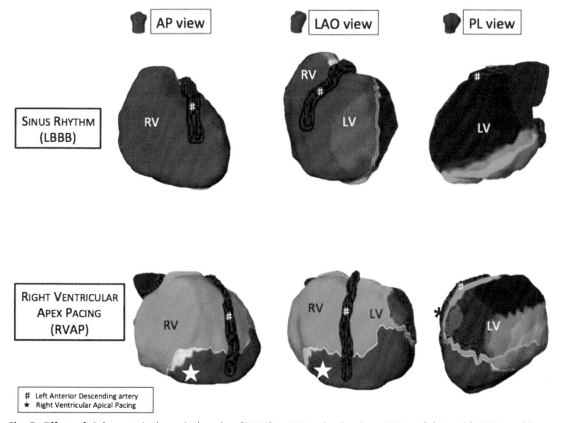

Left Anterior Descending artery
★ Right Ventricular Apical Pacing

Fig. 5. Effect of right ventricular apical pacing (RVAP) on RV activation in a CRT candidate with LBBB and heart failure. During LBBB activation, there is a single lateral RV breakthrough site. During RVAP pacing, as expected, there is an apical RV breakthrough site. During LBBB, RV electrical activation is rapid (full red area) and lines of slow conduction were not observed. In contrast with RVAP pacing, right ventricular propagation seems to occur more slowly, with a curvilinear line of slow conduction observed around the pacing site (border of the red area). As a result, RV total activation time is prolonged during RVAP.[22] Note that LV activation also changes. AP, anteroposterior; LAO, left anterior oblique; PL, posterolateral.[10]

to conduction.[10] This potential advantage for LV preexcitation may be captured by retaining RV pacing, timed with LV activation. However, the advantage of LV pacing may not depend on fusion with intrinsic RBB conduction. Some studies have shown that LV-only stimulation at short AV intervals with complete capture (and wide QRS) resulted in positive outcome, similar to biventricular stimulation.[25,26] This benefit, occurring despite lack of restoration of electrical dyssynchrony, challenges some of the fundamental concepts underlying resynchronization therapy.[26]

Alternative Pacing Sites

There has been considerable interest in alternative pacing sites in both LV and RV. A trend to better preservation of LV function with nonapical RV endocardial pacing sites has been observed.[27]

This trend suggests a potential mechanism and importance of different patterns of LV activation.[10] Whether these promote better resynchronization with LV paced wave fronts during CRT remains unevaluated. In recognition of the potential impediment created by conduction barriers, a strategy of multipolar leads or addition of a separate LV lead to jump conduction block has been tested. However, the modest, if any, benefit observed with these strategies may relate to the lack of electrical guidance by, for example, ECGI to optimize these lead positions. LV endocardial pacing may achieve more than 2-fold faster LV activation compared with epicardial stimulation from the CS.[21] These rapid conduction endocardial tissue planes may be engaged from the RV transseptally.[28] These data indicate the importance of assessing electrical response to pacing for hemodynamic benefit and improved long-term outcome.

Electrocardiographic Activation Map of a Clinical Responder to CRT With a 12-Lead Surface ECG Exhibiting a NICD Activation Pattern

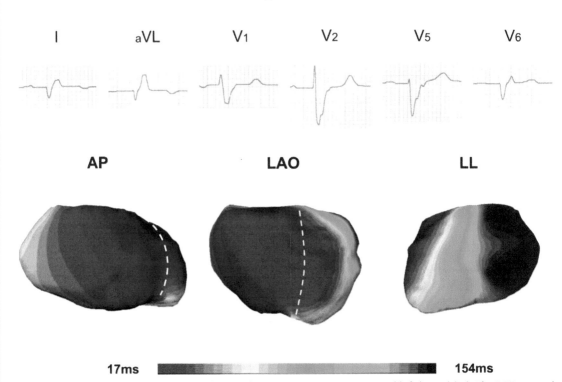

Fig. 6. Epicardial surfaces of both ventricles are shown in 3 views: AP, LAO, and left lateral (LL). The LAD artery is depicted as a white dotted line. On the 12-lead ECG, the QR pattern in lead I and the absence of a broad notched R wave in V5 and V6 are criteria against the diagnosis of LBBB. The right ventricular breakthrough is followed by a fast activation of this ventricle. The wave front spread to the left, crossing a first anterolateral line of slow conduction. There is a second atypical area of slow conduction that is more transverse and nonuniform and allows the lateral base to be activated before its adjacent regions. QRS duration, 167 milliseconds; VEU, 82 milliseconds. (*From* Ploux S, Lumens J, Whinnett Z, et al. Noninvasive electrocardiographic mapping to improve patient selection for cardiac resynchronization therapy: beyond QRS duration and left bundle-branch block morphology. J Am Coll Cardiol 2013;61(24):2440; with permission.)

Non–Left Bundle Branch Block QRS Morphologies

These morphologies represent a heterogeneous group of conduction defects including RBBB and nonspecific intraventricular conduction defects (NICDs). The presence of LV activation delay, if any, is infrequent.[4] Under these circumstances CRT, which usually imposes LV pacing in already-early activated tissue, may be ineffective or even harmful. This possibility has been corroborated by recent large-scale trials.[3] However, treatment of the minority who do have LV activation delays equivalent to those seen with LBBB may be beneficial. We recently showed the importance of the variations in activation sequence and electrical dyssynchrony among patients with NICDs. They usually present a unique RV epicardial breakthrough, but multiple sites of epicardial breakthrough may be seen (including the LV epicardium), lines of slow conduction occur infrequently and tend to be shorter than those seen in LBBB, and the latest activated region is variable. There is a broad spectrum of interventricular delay: LV relative to RV delay may range from negative (indicating RV delay) to greater than 50 milliseconds (ie, LV delay). LV delay may be readily identified by ECGI (**Fig. 6**) and elicits a positive response to biventricular pacing.

SUMMARY

CRT is an electrical therapy that may be best understood by characterization of electrical substrate and its interaction with pacing, which are depicted in only rudimentary fashion by the surface ECG. In contrast, noninvasive ECGI provides high-resolution single-beat ventricular mapping that revealed significant heterogeneity of LV activation in patients with heart failure with QRS prolongation, coupled to unpredictable LV activation in response to LV pacing, even in the absence of scar. These electrical variations may have significant implications for CRT, independently of modulating factors such as ischemic disease and renal failure. This hypothesis merits prospective evaluation in a large-scale trial.

REFERENCES

1. Cleland JG, Daubert JC, Erdmann E, et al. The effect of cardiac resynchronization on morbidity and mortality in heart failure. N Engl J Med 2005; 352(15):1539–49.
2. Chung ES, Leon AR, Tavazzi L, et al. Results of the Predictors of Response to CRT (PROSPECT) trial. Circulation 2008;117(20):2608–16.
3. Zareba W, Klein H, Cygankiewicz I, et al. Effectiveness of cardiac resynchronization therapy by QRS morphology in the multicenter automatic defibrillator implantation trial-cardiac resynchronization therapy (MADIT-CRT). Circulation 2011;123(10):1061–72.
4. Varma N. Left ventricular conduction delays and relation to QRS configuration in patients with left ventricular dysfunction. Am J Cardiol 2009;103: 1578–85.
5. Gold MR, Birgersdotter-Green U, Singh JP, et al. The relationship between ventricular electrical delay and left ventricular remodelling with cardiac resynchronization therapy. Eur Heart J 2011;32(20):2516–24.
6. Varma N, Manne M, Nguyen D, et al. Probability and magnitude of response to cardiac resynchronization therapy according to QRS duration and gender in nonischemic cardiomyopathy and LBBB. Heart Rhythm 2014;11(7):1139–47.
7. Ramanathan C, Ghanem RN, Jia P, et al. Noninvasive electrocardiographic imaging for cardiac electrophysiology and arrhythmia. Nat Med 2004;10(4): 422–8.
8. Ramanathan C, Jia P, Ghanem R, et al. Activation and repolarization of the normal human heart under complete physiological conditions. Proc Natl Acad Sci U S A 2006;103(16):6309–14.
9. Auricchio A, Fantoni C, Regoli F, et al. Characterization of left ventricular activation in patients with heart failure and left bundle-branch block. Circulation 2004;109(9):1133–9.
10. Varma N. Left ventricular electrical activation during right ventricular pacing in heart failure patients with LBBB: visualization by electrocardiographic imaging and implications for cardiac resynchronization therapy. J Electrocardiol 2014. [Epub ahead of print].
11. Tse HF, Lee KL, Wan SH, et al. Area of left ventricular regional conduction delay and preserved myocardium predict responses to cardiac resynchronization therapy. J Cardiovasc Electrophysiol 2005; 16(7):690–5.
12. Kanzaki H, Bazaz R, Schwartzman D, et al. A mechanism for immediate reduction in mitral regurgitation after cardiac resynchronization therapy: insights from mechanical activation strain mapping. J Am Coll Cardiol 2004;44(8):1619–25.
13. Jia P, Ramanathan C, Ghanem RN, et al. Electrocardiographic imaging of cardiac resynchronization therapy in heart failure: observation of variable electrophysiologic responses. Heart Rhythm 2006;3(3): 296–310.
14. Ghosh S, Avari JN, Rhee EK, et al. Noninvasive electrocardiographic imaging (ECGI) of epicardial activation before and after catheter ablation of the accessory pathway in a patient with Ebstein anomaly. Heart Rhythm 2008;5(6):857–60.
15. Ploux S, Lumens J, Whinnett Z, et al. Noninvasive electrocardiographic mapping to improve patient

selection for cardiac resynchronization therapy: beyond QRS duration and left bundle-branch block morphology. J Am Coll Cardiol 2013;61(24):2435–43.

16. Leyva F, Foley PW, Chalil S, et al. Cardiac resynchronization therapy guided by late gadolinium-enhancement cardiovascular magnetic resonance. J Cardiovasc Magn Reson 2011;13:29.

17. Varma N. Cardiac resynchronization therapy and the electrical substrate in heart failure: what does the QRS conceal? Heart Rhythm 2009;6:1059–62.

18. Lambiase PD, Rinaldi A, Hauck J, et al. Non-contact left ventricular endocardial mapping in cardiac resynchronisation therapy. Heart 2004;90(1):44–51.

19. Varma N, Jia P, Rudy Y. Placebo CRT. J Cardiovasc Electrophysiol 2008;19(8):878.

20. Dekker AL, Phelps B, Dijkman B, et al. Epicardial left ventricular lead placement for cardiac resynchronization therapy: optimal pace site selection with pressure-volume loops. J Thorac Cardiovasc Surg 2004;127(6):1641–7.

21. Derval N, Steendijk P, Gula LJ, et al. Optimizing hemodynamics in heart failure patients by systematic screening of left ventricular pacing sites: the lateral left ventricular wall and the coronary sinus are rarely the best sites. J Am Coll Cardiol 2010;55(6):566–75.

22. Varma N, Jia P, Ramanathan C, et al. RV electrical activation in heart failure during right, left, and biventricular pacing. JACC Cardiovasc Imaging 2010; 3(6):567–75.

23. Lee KL, Burnes JE, Mullen TJ, et al. Avoidance of right ventricular pacing in cardiac resynchronization therapy improves right ventricular hemodynamics in heart failure patients. J Cardiovasc Electrophysiol 2007;18(5):497–504.

24. Martin DO, Lemke B, Birnie D, et al. Investigation of a novel algorithm for synchronized left-ventricular pacing and ambulatory optimization of cardiac resynchronization therapy: results of the adaptive CRT trial. Heart Rhythm 2012;9(11):1807–14.

25. Thibault B, Ducharme A, Harel F, et al. Left ventricular versus simultaneous biventricular pacing in patients with heart failure and a QRS complex >/= 120 milliseconds. Circulation 2011;124(25):2874–81.

26. Lumens J, Ploux S, Strik M, et al. Comparative electromechanical and hemodynamic effects of left ventricular and biventricular pacing in dyssynchronous heart failure: electrical resynchronization versus left-right ventricular interaction. J Am Coll Cardiol 2013;62(25):2395–403.

27. Shimony A, Eisenberg MJ, Filion KB, et al. Beneficial effects of right ventricular non-apical vs. apical pacing: a systematic review and meta-analysis of randomized-controlled trials. Europace 2012;14(1): 81–91.

28. Strik M, Rademakers LM, van Deursen CJ, et al. Endocardial left ventricular pacing improves cardiac resynchronization therapy in chronic asynchronous infarction and heart failure models. Circ Arrhythm Electrophysiol 2012;5(1):191–200.

29. Durrer D, van Dam RT, Freud GE, et al. Total excitation of the isolated human heart. Circulation 1970; 41(6):899–912.

Pediatric Electrocardiographic Imaging Applications

Jennifer N.A. Silva, MD

KEYWORDS

- Electrocardiographic imaging • Pediatrics • Congenital heart disease • Wolff–Parkinson–White
- Cardiac resynchronization therapy

KEY POINTS

- Noninvasive electrocardiographic imaging (ECGI) provides clinically useful information in the pediatric and congenital heart disease populations.
- Pediatric ECGI can be performed safely in young patients.
- ECGI can be used to localize the site of accessory pathways in patients with structurally normal hearts, congenital heart disease, and cardiomyopathy.
- ECGI may provide important data in patients before, during, and after cardiac resynchronization therapy.

INTRODUCTION

Electrocardiographic imaging (ECGI) is a novel noninvasive imaging modality used to study the electrophysiologic substrate in patients. This tool has also been successfully applied to pediatric patients, some as young as 18 months of age, to create patient-specific models of atrial and ventricular activation and repolarization. In this article, we review the pediatric applications of ECGI and what these studies have contributed the general knowledge of pediatric electrophysiology.

MANIFEST ACCESSORY PATHWAY IN A PATIENT WITH EBSTEIN'S ANOMALY

Ebstein's anomaly is a rare congenital heart disease involving the septal and posterior leaflets of the tricuspid valve, where the leaflets may be deformed, displaced, or adherent to the intraventricular septum.[1] Patients are prone to electrical problems as well, with up to 25% having concomitant preexcitation on surface 12-lead electrocardiograms. Arrhythmic substrates in these patients include supraventricular tachycardia, atrial flutter and atrial fibrillation. Accessory pathways (APs) are typically single pathways localized to the right-sided Ebstenoid tricuspid valve.

ECGI was performed in this patient to construct ventricular activation maps before and after ablation, as well as postablation potential maps.

Methods and Results

A 16-year-old with Ebstein's anomaly and ventricular preexcitation underwent ECGI to construct ventricular activation maps during a single preexcited beat before ablation.[1] Applying the Arruda algorithm[2] to the baseline preablation, preexcited ECG (**Fig. 1**), the delta wave mapped the AP to a subepicardial/right posteroseptal location.

ECGI was performed during 2 time points, before and after ablation. **Fig. 2** demonstrates the preablation activation isochronal map (see **Fig. 2**A, B), postablation activation map (see **Fig. 2**C, D) and

The author has nothing to disclose.
Division of Pediatric Cardiology, Washington University School of Medicine, 1 Children's Place, Campus Box 8116, Saint Louis, MO 63110, USA
E-mail address: silva_j@kids.wustl.edu

Card Electrophysiol Clin 7 (2015) 135–152
http://dx.doi.org/10.1016/j.ccep.2014.11.006

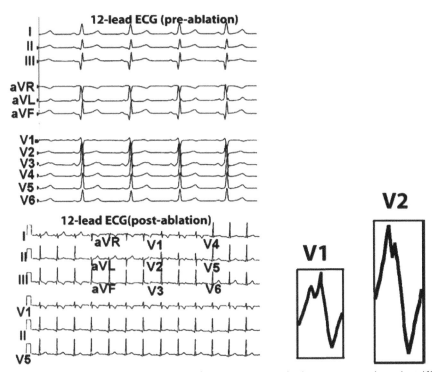

Fig. 1. These preablation and postablation ECGs are from a patient with Ebstein's anomaly and Wolff–Parkinson–White syndrome. On the upper panel, before ablation, note the positive delta wave in lead I and negative delta waves in leads II and III, indicating a subepicardial/right posteroseptal location of the AP per the Arruda algorithm. In the bottom panel, after ablation, there are no longer delta waves present and there is a notched R wave in leads V1 and V2 with a QRS duration of 90 ms. (*From* Ghosh S, Avari JN, Rhee RK, et al. Noninvasive electrocardiographic imaging (ECGI) of epicardial activation before and after catheter ablation of the accessory pathway in a patient with Ebstein anomaly. Heart Rhythm 2008;5(6):858; with permission.)

the postablation potential maps (see **Fig. 2**E, F) in the right anterior oblique projection (see **Fig. 2**A, C, E) and the left lateral projections (see **Fig. 2**B, D, F). In the preablation isochronal maps, the earliest site of ventricular activation (area of red) is localized to the right posterolateral location on the tricuspid valve annulus as marked by the white asterisk (see **Fig. 2**A). Ventricular activation then propagates in a uniform manner with the left ventricle (LV) activating late (areas of blue; see **Fig. 2**B).

The following day, the patient underwent an electrophysiology study (EPS) and transcatheter ablation. A 3-dimensional electroanatomic map was created (CARTO, Biosense Webster, Diamond Bar, CA, USA) to localize the AP. **Fig. 3**A shows the earliest site of activation identified in the right posterolateral region of the tricuspid valve annulus, similar to where ECGI had predicted the pathway location. A cryocatheter was positioned at the site of the AP (see **Fig. 3**B) there was cessation of AP activity within 8 seconds of initiating cryotherapy.

Postablation ECGI images were obtained (see **Fig. 2**C, D) and showed the activation in the right posterolateral region to now be late (area of blue;

marked by the + sign). The earliest ventricular activation after ablation is now in the anterior paraseptal region and inferior anteroapical region of the right ventricle (RV).

Fig. 2E, F shows the ECGI epicardial potential map postablation (at 38 ms after QRS). A local minimum potential (area of blue, marked by black asterisk) is seen on the anterior RV surface midway between the RV base and the left anterior descending artery indicating RV breakthrough. This site of RV breakthrough occurs at 38 ms after QRS onset and 13 ms after earliest LV epicardial breakthrough. Conduction throughout the RV is slow with the right ventricular outflow tract being the latest to activate. Activation of the LV occurs in the normal apex to base with the basal posterolateral area being the last to activate (area of blue, **Fig. 2**D).

Summary

During normal ventricular activation, the earliest area of epicardial activation occurs on the anterior RV (18–20 ms after the QRS), indicating normal conduction and function of the right

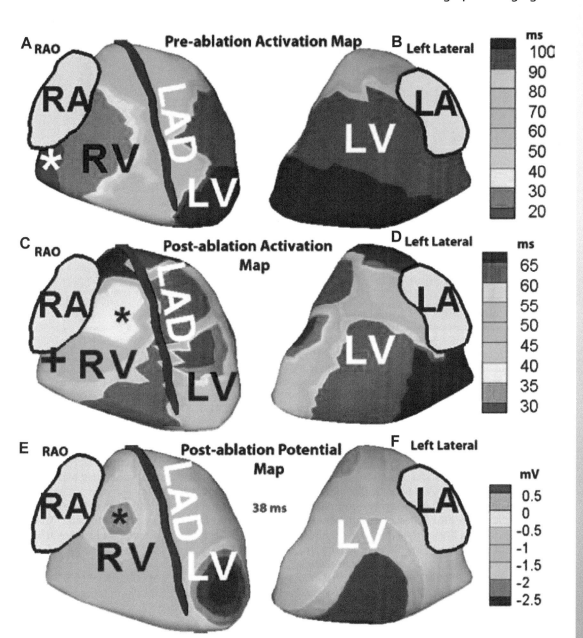

Fig. 2. The right anterior oblique (RAO) and left lateral projections during 3 time points are shown in this patient with Ebstein's anomaly and Wolff–Parkinson–White syndrome. (*A, B*) Ventricular activation isochronal maps obtained before ablation. (*C, D*) Ventricular isochronal activation maps obtained after ablation. The earliest right ventricular breakthrough (RVBT) is marked by a black asterisk (*C,E*). (*E, F*) Postablation potential map obtained 38 ms after the onset of surface QRS complex. LA, left atrium; LAD, left anterior descending; LV, left ventricle; RA, right atrium; RV, right ventricle. (*From* Ghosh S, Avari JN, Rhee RK, et al. Noninvasive electrocardiographic imaging (ECGI) of epicardial activation before and after catheter ablation of the accessory pathway in a patient with Ebstein anomaly. Heart Rhythm 2008;5(6):858; with permission.)

bundle branch. This is followed by additional RV epicardial breakthrough sites, resulting in a synchronized contraction. Epicardial LV activation occurs next, about 10 ms after RV epicardial breakthrough. In this case, however, RV breakthrough after ablation lags behind the LV breakthrough, occurring 13 ms after LV breakthrough

and 38 ms after QRS onset (see **Fig. 2**C). On the postablation potential map (see **Fig. 2**E), we see a site of potential minimum (black asterisk) near the site of RV epicardial breakthrough (see **Fig. 2**C).

However, the delayed appearance of the RV breakthrough (38 ms after QRS, 12 ms after LV

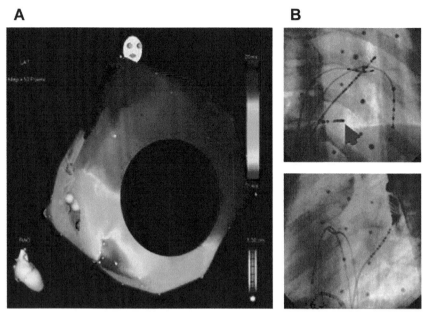

Fig. 3. Images obtained during the invasive electrophysiologic study in a patient with Ebstein's anomaly and Wolff–Parkinson–White syndrome. (*A*) Three-dimensional electroanatomic map (CARTO map) of the tricuspid valve annulus that demonstrates the area of earliest activation along the right posterolateral region. (*B*) Ablation catheter (CryoCatheter; distal tip marked by red arrow) at the site of ablation success, in the right anterior oblique (RAO; *top panel*) and left anterior oblique (LAO; *bottom panel*) views. This catheter location correlates with the location predicted by ECGI in **Fig. 1**A, B. (*Adapted from* Ghosh S, Avari JN, Rhee RK, et al. Noninvasive electrocardiographic imaging (ECGI) of epicardial activation before and after catheter ablation of the accessory pathway in a patient with Ebstein anomaly. Heart Rhythm 2008;5(6):859; with permission.)

breakthrough) suggests that the conduction through the right bundle branch is slower compared with normal. Additionally, the paraseptal and apical areas of the RV are late to activate (areas of blue, see **Fig. 2**C) supporting slow RV bundle conduction. This is reflected in the surface ECG after ablation (see **Fig. 1**), where there are notched R waves in leads V1 and V2 with a QRS duration of 90 ms. ECGI demonstrated that this finding on the surface ECG represented true slow conduction through the RV bundle branch.

The patient underwent successful ablation of a single AP in the posterolateral aspect of the tricuspid valve annulus. ECGI successfully predicted the pathway location. Patients with congenital heart disease highlight the inaccuracies of standard, noninvasive AP localization algorithms, such as the Arruda algorithm. ECGI, which incorporates patient-specific heart–torso geometry with electrophysiologic properties, provides more accuracy in AP localization.

PEDIATRIC HYPERTROPHIC CARDIOMYOPATHY WITH VENTRICULAR PREEXCITATION

Hypertrophic cardiomyopathy (HCM) accounts for 42% of all childhood cardiomyopathies with an incidence of 0.47 in 100,000 children.[3,4] It is defined as the presence of ventricular hypertrophy without an identifiable cause.

This is the case of an 18-year-old male patient with HCM with no history of arrhythmias.[3] The patient's echocardiogram revealed significant HCM (septal thickness of 2.17 cm, Z-score 7.5, with LV posterior wall thickness of 1.43 cm, z-score 3.6) with no evidence of LV outflow tract obstruction. Twelve-lead ECG demonstrated manifest preexcitation with delta wave map (by Arruda algorithm[2]) prediction of a right anteroseptal AP.

Methods and Results

ECGI epicardial activation maps were created during preexcited sinus rhythm (**Fig. 4**). **Fig. 4**A demonstrates the earliest area of activation was localized to the right anterior/anteroseptal region (area of white) of the tricuspid valve annulus. Additionally, the midseptal region and right posteroseptal regions were also early (areas of pink). The entire LV basal area (area of red) was also activated early. Activation spread from base to apex (see **Fig. 4**C) in a uniform manner with an elongated area of early activation in the RV along the interventricular groove. In normal (nonpreexcited) sinus rhythm, this area is typically the

Epicardial Activation Map (HCM and Pre-excitation)

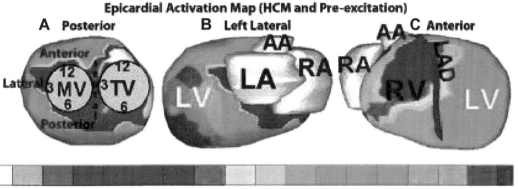

Epicardial Activation Map (Normal)

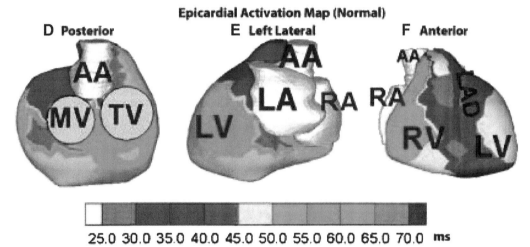

Fig. 4. Electrocardiographic imaging–generated epicardial activation maps obtained in a patient with hypertrophic cardiomyopathy and preexcitation (*top row*), in a posterior, left lateral, and anterior projections. The second row demonstrates the epicardial activation maps from a normal healthy male for comparison. AA, ascending aorta; HCM, hypertrophic cardiomyopathy; LA, left atrium; LAD, left anterior descending; LV, left ventricle; MV, mitral valve; RA, right atrium; RV, right ventricle; TV, tricuspid valve. (*From* Ghosh S, Avari JN, Rhee EK, et al. Hypertrophic cardiomyopathy with preexcitation: insights from noninvasive electrocardiographic imaging (ECGI) and catheter mapping. J Cardiovasc Electrophysiol 2008;19(11):1216; with permission.)

earliest area of epicardial activation; however, in the face of this patient's preexcitation syndrome, activation in this region was 26 ms later than the right anteroseptal location (see **Fig. 4**D–F, which demonstrate epicardial ventricular activation in a healthy, nonpreexcited 21-year-old male. Areas of early epicardial activation occur in the RV along the interventricular groove with uniform activation spreading throughout the ventricles, with the left posterobasal area being last to activate.)

This patient underwent EPS the following day. Initial intervals demonstrated a short His-Ventricular interval at 12 ms. With atrial extrastimulus testing, there was no change in the QRS morphology despite AH decrement. The shortest

preexcited RR interval with atrial overdrive pacing was 320 ms, after which Wenckebach occurred. Atrial pacing was performed from multiple sites in both the right and left atria with no change in QRS morphology. Intravenous adenosine was administered, which showed PR prolongation with no augmentation of preexcitation (no change in QRS). Ventricular pacing demonstrated no retrograde conduction. Activation mapping found a fragmented multiphasic His recording at the 2:30 position along the tricuspid valve annulus with a local activation time of -18 ms before the delta wave (**Fig. 5**). No tachyarrhythmias were induced throughout the study. These findings were consistent with a fasiculoventricular pathway.

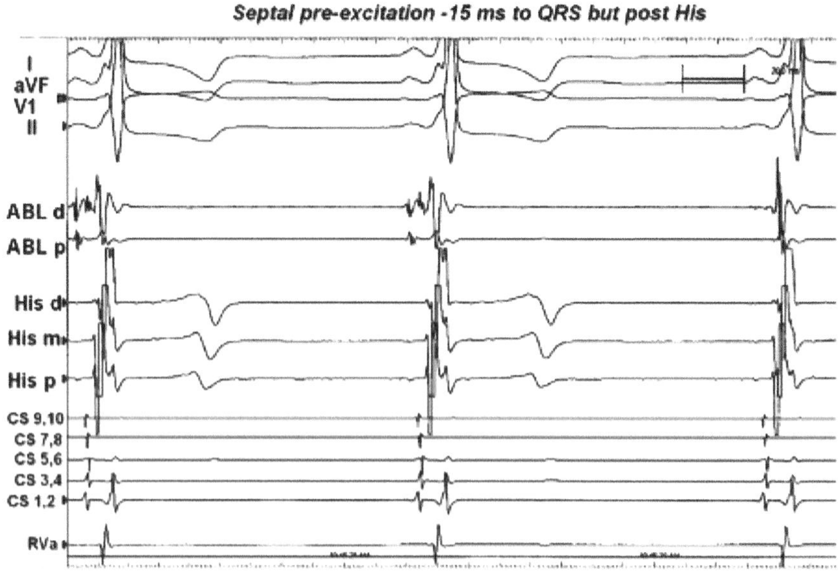

Fig. 5. Intracardiac signals from an electrophysiology study performed in a patient with hypertrophic cardiomyopathy and preexcitation. The ablation catheter has been placed in the area of earliest ventricular activation and shows that there is septal preexcitation (measuring 15 ms before QRS), but it comes after the His signal. (*From* Ghosh S, Avari JN, Rhee EK, et al. Hypertrophic cardiomyopathy with preexcitation: insights from noninvasive electrocardiographic imaging (ECGI) and catheter mapping. J Cardiovasc Electrophysiol 2008;19(11):1215; with permission.)

Summary

Despite the abnormal activation sequence generated by ECGI mapping, the EPS confirmed the presence of a fasiculoventricular pathway that did not mediate supraventricular tachycardia. The septal preexcitation without inducible tachycardia may be attributed to enhanced conduction via a "short" bundle branch, or alternatively, a fasiculoventricular pathway. The presence of asymptomatic preexcitation in a patient with HCM should raise the suspicion of a fasiculoventricular pathway.

CARDIAC MEMORY IN PEDIATRIC WOLFF–PARKINSON–WHITE PATIENTS

Cardiac memory is the phenomenon of repolarization changes induced by long-standing, altered cardiac activation (eg, pacing) which persist for a period of time after normal activation has been restored.[5] The mechanism of cardiac memory is a remodeling process that alters molecular determinants of the action potential duration, such as membrane density and kinetic properties of ion channels.

Wolff–Parkinson–White syndrome involves long-standing altered activation sequence owing to ventricular preexcitation and provides a "natural model" for studying cardiac memory. Ablation of the AP with the restoration of sinus rhythm provides a model for understanding the time course of repolarization changes.

Objectives of this study were to (1) utilize ECGI for the localization of AP location in patients with Wolff–Parkinson–White syndrome and (2) image activation and repolarization before and at several time points after ablation to study the time course of activation and repolarization changes, or cardiac memory.[5]

Methods and Results

Fourteen pediatric patients with Wolff–Parkinson–White syndrome and structurally normal hearts referred for EPS and transcatheter ablation were enrolled in this study. Patients underwent ECGI before ablation, 45 minutes after ablation (in sinus rhythm), and at 1 week and 1 month after ablation.

In **Fig. 6**, there are preablation epicardial potential maps in the first column and ventricular activation maps in the second column. Patient W1 (top row) has the earliest epicardial breakthrough (see **Fig. 6**A) indicated by a deep local potential minimum in the posterior septum on the left atrioventricular (AV) valve (AVV) annulus, at the 7 o'clock position (area of dark blue). This was seen 8 ms after the onset of the delta-wave on surface ECG. The epicardial potential map during repolarization, 181 ms after the onset of delta wave (see **Fig. 6**B) showed a similar albeit reversed pattern as activation with the minimum now replaced by a potential

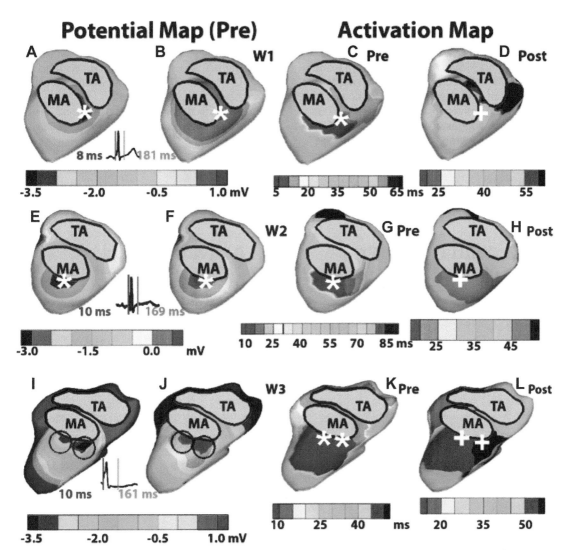

Fig. 6. Electrocardiographic imaging maps for patients W1, W2, and W3. Maps in the first column of are activation and repolarization potential maps before ablation. In the second column, there are ventricular activation maps before and after ablation. Initiation site marked by asterisk. In the bottom row, black circles mark the two discrete potential minima (*I*) and maxima (*J*). Preablation preexcitation region marked by plus symbols. MA, mitral annulus; TA, tricuspid annulus. (*From* Ghosh S, Rhee EK, Avari JN, et al. Cardiac memory in patients with Wolff–Parkinson–White syndrome: noninvasive imaging of activation and repolarization before and after catheter ablation. Circulation 2008;26:118(9):909; with permission.)

maximum. The preablation ventricular activation map (see **Fig. 6**C) shows early ventricular activation at the same location indicating the location of the AP. Postablation ECGI isochrones map shows late activation in the left posterior area of the mitral valve annulus with the latest area of activation on the right AVV annulus, in the posterolateral region.

Patient W2 in **Fig. 6** illustrates a left lateral pathway. The epicardial potential map shows a deep potential minimum in the left lateral aspect of the mitral valve (see **Fig. 6**E) with the repolarization potential map (see **Fig. 6**F) showing the inverse, a

positive potential at the same location. In **Fig. 6**G, the preablation ventricular activation map localizes the AP location to the left lateral AVV annulus. After ablation, the site of the former AP is now an area of late activation.

The epicardial activation potential map in patient W3 (see **Fig. 6**I) shows 2 discrete sites of epicardial potential minima (circled areas), one in a left lateral location and one in a more posterolateral location. The epicardial repolarization potential map (see **Fig. 6**J) shows the same 2 discrete maxima at the same locations where we saw the minima during activation. The preablation activation map (see

Fig. 6K) demonstrated a broad area of early activation encompassing the same region as denoted on the potential maps. During the ablation procedure, there were 2 confirmed AP targets located—one on the left lateral aspect and one on the left posterolateral aspect of the left AVV. The presence of the 2 minima during activation, and the 2 maxima during repolarization suggested the presence of 2 APs. Postablation isochrones indicated late areas of activation at the left lateral and posterolateral locations.

In Fig. 7 (patient W4), we see an example of a patient with a right posteroseptal AP. ECGI activation

(see Fig. 7A) and repolarization (see Fig. 7B) potential maps, as well as preablation activation map, localized the AP site to near the mouth of the coronary sinus. The postablation activation map (see Fig. 7D) showed an area of late activation in the right posterior septum.

Patient W5 in Fig. 7 has an AP that demonstrates potential breakthrough (see Fig. 7E) and early activation (see Fig. 7G) in the midseptal area. For this location, ECGI was not able to determine laterality of the pathway (right vs left midseptal) because the reconstructions are limited to the epicardial surface.

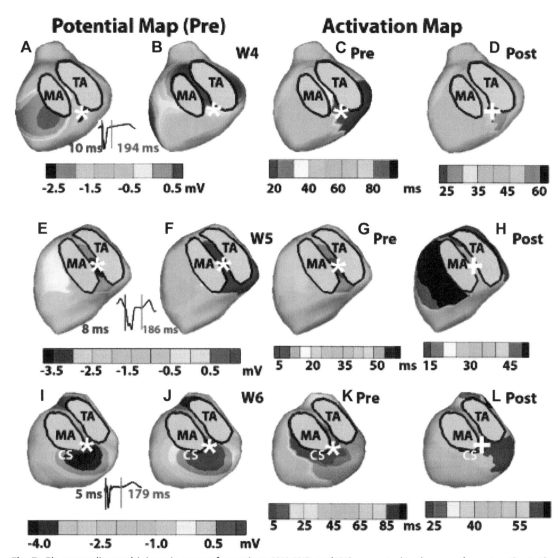

Fig. 7. Electrocardiographic imaging maps for patients W4, W5, and W6 presented in the same format as Fig. 6. The first column shows activation and repolarization potential maps before ablation. In the second column are ventricular activation maps before and after ablation. MA, mitral annulus; TA, tricuspid annulus. (From Ghosh S, Rhee EK, Avari JN, et al. Cardiac memory in patients with Wolff–Parkinson–White syndrome: noninvasive imaging of activation and repolarization before and after catheter ablation. Circulation 2008;26:118(9):911; with permission.)

Patient W6 in **Fig. 7** had epicardial activation (see **Fig. 7I**) and repolarization (see **Fig. 7J**) potential maps in the left posteroseptal region. Preablation and postablation epicardial activation maps (see **Fig. 7K, L**) also confirmed this finding.

For 5 patients, ECGI maps of retrograde atrial activation were generated when clear retrograde P waves were visible on the body surface ECG. **Fig. 8** shows 2 representative examples of these maps. For patient W1 (**Fig. 8**, top row), the retrograde atrial activation patterns during sustained tachycardia are shown in **Fig. 8A, B**. The earliest area of activation, in white, is localized to the left posterior atrial wall. Activation then spread in a uniform fashion from this location throughout the atria, with the low anterior right atria activating last (blue).

In **Fig. 8**, second row, we see the retrograde atrial activation for patient W5 who had a right sided midseptal AP. The area of earliest retrograde activation occurs in the lower right atrium, through the right atrium, and to the posterior aspect of the atria, with the lateral left atrium/left atrial appendage being the last to activate.

Antegrade ventricular activation is demonstrated in patients W1 and W5 in **Fig. 8**. There was early antegrade ventricular activation in the RV in the apical (W1) and paraseptal (W5) regions, with late activation in the posterolateral RV (W1) or left lateral basilar area (W5). ECGI ventricular activation maps during supraventricular tachycardia were found to be similar to normal sinus (nonpreexcited) rhythm maps, indicating that antegrade conduction involved the AV node/His–Purkinje system.

Figs. 9 and **10** show ECGI epicardial activation-recovery interval (ARI) maps that were generated at 4 distinct time points: (1) before ablation, (2) 45 minutes after ablation, (3) 1 week after ablation, and (4) 1 month after ablation. In patients W1 through W5, the epicardial electrogram at the site of the AP demonstrated a rS morphology, indicating an endocardial insertion site of the AP. In patient W6, however, the epicardial electrogram at the AP site demonstrated a pure QS morphology, indicating the insertion site of the AP to be epicardial or subepicardial. Additionally, the T waves for patients

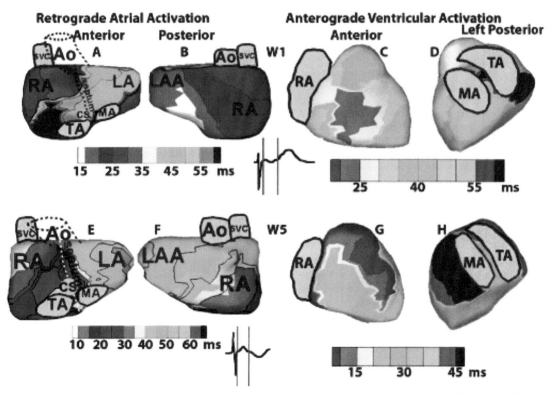

Fig. 8. Electrocardiographic imaging–generated maps during sustained supraventricular tachycardia of retrograde atrial activation (*first column*) and antegrade ventricular activation (*second column*) in 2 patients, W1 and W5. Inset, Lead V$_2$ of ECG during SVT, with the red lines marking the start and end of the retrograde P wave after the QRS complex. Ao, aorta; CS, coronary sinus; LA, left atrium; LAA, left ascending aorta; MA, mitral annulus; RA, right atrium; SVC, superior vena cava; TA, tricuspid annulus. (*From* Ghosh S, Rhee EK, Avari JN, et al. Cardiac memory in patients with Wolff–Parkinson–White syndrome: noninvasive imaging of activation and repolarization before and after catheter ablation. Circulation 2008;26:118(9):912; with permission.)

Activation-Recovery Interval (ARI) Maps

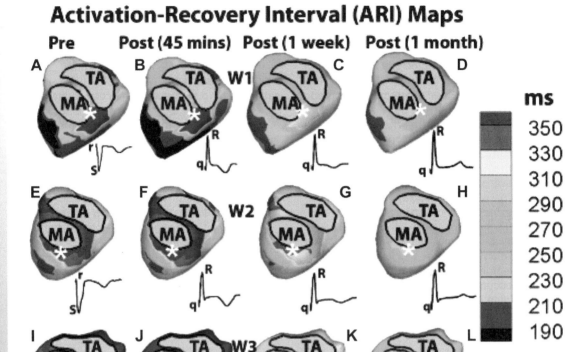

Fig. 9. Activation recovery interval maps of patients W1, W2, and W3 created before, after, and at 1 week and 1 month after ablation. The inset in each panel shows the noninvasively reconstructed epicardial electrogram from the preablation site of earliest preexcitation (*asterisk*). MA, mitral annulus; TA, tricuspid annulus. (*From* Ghosh S, Rhee EK, Avari JN, et al. Cardiac memory in patients with Wolff–Parkinson–White syndrome: noninvasive imaging of activation and repolarization before and after catheter ablation. Circulation 2008;26:118(9):912; with permission.)

W1-W6 before ablation were inverted (see **Figs. 9** and **10**A, E, I).

The ARI maps at 45 minutes after ablation (see **Figs. 9** and **10**B, F, J) demonstrated a change in the epicardial electrogram morphology from a rS (or QS) to a qR pattern, with persistent inversion of the T waves. By 1 week after ablation, the T waves remained inverted, although to a lesser extent, and finally became more flattened and upright by 1 month after ablation.

The basilar annular region had the highest ARI in preexcited rhythm (see **Figs. 9** and **10**A, E, I) with the area of longest ARIs at the preexcitation site. This ARI distribution was largely unchanged at 45 minutes after ablation. By 1 week after ablation, the ARI decreased but remained high. At 1 month after ablation, the ARI has normalized.

In **Table 1**, the predicted site of the AP by ECGI is compared with the predicted site using the Arruda algorithm. The site of successful ablation is also shown. ECGI localization was fairly accurate to site of ablation success, within a 1-hour arc along the annulus.

Summary

ECGI is able to predict accurately and precisely the site of APs. Additionally, ECGI was able to predict epicardial versus endocardial location, as well as multiple Aps, thus distinguishing it from noninvasive algorithms created to predict AP location.

Abnormal repolarization in patients with Wolff–Parkinson–White syndrome results in altered epicardial apical–basal ARI dispersion. Although activation patterns normalize immediately upon ablation of the manifest AP, repolarization patterns remain abnormal and unchanged. At 1 week after ablation, we see that the recovery gradients are still abnormal but have gradually decreased and have normalized by 1 month after ablation. This

Activation-Recovery Interval (ARI) Maps

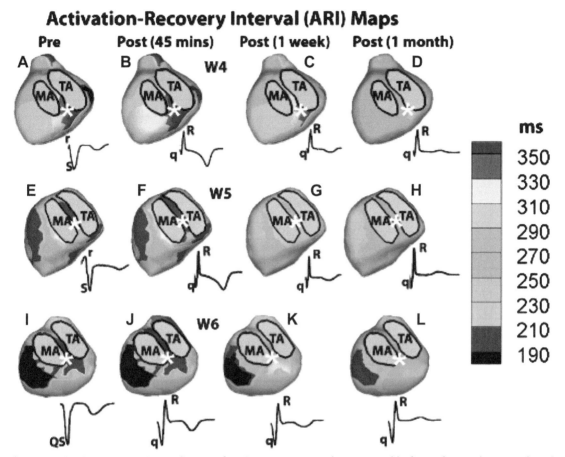

Fig. 10. Activation-recovery interval maps of patients W4, W5, and W6 created before, after, and at 1 week and 1 month after ablation presented in the same format as **Fig. 9**. (*From* Ghosh S, Rhee EK, Avari JN, et al. Cardiac memory in patients with Wolff–Parkinson–White syndrome: noninvasive imaging of activation and repolarization before and after catheter ablation. Circulation 2008;26:118(9):913; with permission.)

time course is consistent with the phenomenon of cardiac memory.

CARDIAC RESYNCHRONIZATION THERAPY IN PEDIATRIC CONGENITAL HEART DISEASE PATIENTS

Cardiac resynchronization therapy (CRT) has been studied extensively in adult heart failure patients; it has been less thoroughly studied in children and congenital heart disease patients.[6] Patients with congenital heart disease have been living longer owing to improvements in surgical management of these patients, and are evolving into young adults with heart failure. CRT has been shown to be advantageous for certain disease substrates.

In this study, there were 3 distinct hypotheses involving ECGI in pediatric CHD: (1) to identify those CHD patients with substantial electrical dyssynchrony in baseline rhythm who would therefore likely benefit from CRT, (2) to help guide the lead

placement of the resynchronization lead by identifying the electrophysiologic substrate and the area of latest activation, and (3) to evaluate intraventricular dyssynchrony after CRT.[6]

Methods and Results

Patients were included if they were (1) less than 21 years old, (2) had congenital heart disease, (3) had heart failure symptoms despite maximized medical therapy, and (4) undergoing evaluation for CRT or having a CRT device in place. ECGI was performed in these patients in the baseline presenting rhythm. For pre-CRT patients who had a pacemaker in place and were not pacemaker dependent, ECGI was also performed in nonpaced rhythm. For post-CRT patients, testing was performed under the following conditions: (1) optimal CRT (CRT-OPT) settings (including the optimal intraventricular, or V-V, delay as determined by referring physician), (2) nominal CRT (CRT-NOM) settings (which refers to the baseline

Table 1
Patient characteristics in a study of cardiac memory in patients with Wolff–Parkinson–White syndrome

Patient	Age (y)	Gender	ECGI Prediction of AP Location	Arruda Prediction of AP Location	Site of Successful Ablation
W1	12	F	MA/7:00/endocardial	LAL/LL	MA/7:00/endocardial
W2	16	M	MA/4:00/endocardial	LAL/LL	MA/4:00/endocardial
W3	5	M	2 APs/MA/3:00 and 5:00/ endocardial	LAL/LL	2 APs/MA/3:00 and 5:00/ endocardial
W4	13	M	TA/5:00/endocardial	PSTA/PSMA	TA/5:00/endocardial
W5	12	F	Either TA 4:00 or MA 8:00/endocardial	PSTA/PSMA	TA/3:00/endocardial
W6	13	M	MA/7:00/epicardial	PSTA	MA/7:00/MCV, epicardial
W7	8	F	MA/7:00/endocardial	LPL/LP	MA/7:00/epicardial
W8	13	F	Either TA 3:00 or MA 9:00/endocardial	PSTA/PSMA	TA/3:00/endocardial
W9	10	M	MA/7:00/endocardial	LPL/LP	MA/7:00/endocardial
W10	15	M	MA/6:00/endocardial	LPL/LP	MA/6:00/endocardial
W11	13	F	TA/6:00/endocardial	RP/RPL	TA/6:00/endocardial
W12	12	F	MA/3:00/endocardial	LL/LAL	MA/3:00/endocardial
W13	12	F	MA/5:00/endocardial	LAL/LL	MA/5:00/endocardial
W14	10	F	TA/5:00/epicardial	MCV/venous anomaly	TA/5:00/CS diverticulum, epicardial

Abbreviations: AP, accessory pathway; ECGI, electrocardiographic imaging; LAL, left anterolateral; LL, left lateral; LP, left posterior; LPL, left posterolateral; MA, mitral annulus; MCV, middle cardiac vein; PSMA, posteroseptal mitral annulus; PSTA, posteroseptal tricuspid annulus; RP, right posterior; RPL, right posterolateral; TA, tricuspid annulus.

Adapted from Ghosh S, Rhee EK, Avari JN, et al. Cardiac memory in patients with Wolff–Parkinson–White syndrome: noninvasive imaging of activation and repolarization before and after catheter ablation. Circulation 2008;26:118(9):907–15.

factory setting of LV ahead of RV by 4 ms), (3) single site ventricular pacing (either RV or LV), and (4) underlying rhythm (where applicable).

An electrical dyssynchrony index (ED, measured in ms) was calculated from activation isochrones as the standard deviation of activation times at 500 discrete epicardial sites of the systemic ventricle. This measures the degree of dyssynchrony of electrical activation across the systemic ventricle (**Table 2**). Normal values were calculated from control patients.

Table 2
Electrical dyssynchrony index

Electrical Dyssynchrony (ms)	Value
<24	Normal
24–28	Mild dyssynchrony
28–32	Moderate dyssynchrony
>32	Severe dyssynchrony

Data from Silva JN, Ghosh S, Bowman TM, et al. Cardiac resynchronization therapy in pediatric congenital heart disease: insights from noninvasive electrocardiographic imaging. Heart Rhythm 2009;6(8):1178–85.

Pre-cardiac resynchronization therapy electrocardiographic imaging patients

Four patients were evaluated with ECGI as part of their pre-CRT evaluation (**Fig. 11**). Patients 1 and 2 had relatively normal ED indices; CRT was deferred in these patients and they were optimized on medical with or without single site pacing (for patient 2) therapy with clinical improvement. Patient 1 has an ED of 22.4 ms with synchronous LV activation. The area of late (in dark blue) us seen near the RV base and is consistent with a right bundle branch block pattern. Patient 2 had ECGI performed in a dual chamber paced rhythm (ventricular lead in the RV lateral apical free wall) and demonstrated an ED on 20.5 ms. Patient 3 had an ED of 28.4 ms, consistent with moderate dyssynchrony. This patient was treated with medication and had resultant clinical improvement, so CRT was deferred. Patient 4 had a severely dyssynchronous systemic ventricle (ED of 37 ms). This patient was optimized on medical

Pre-CRT ECGI Activation-Isochrones

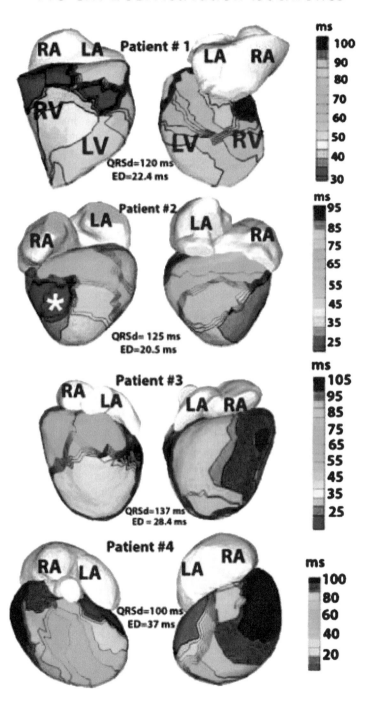

Fig. 11. Electrocardiographic imaging (ECGI) activation isochronal maps from pre-cardiac resynchronization therapy (CRT) patients 1 through 4. The left column projects the heart in an anterior 4-chamber view, and the right column projects the heart in an inferior 4-chamber view. Activation maps were obtained in normal sinus rhythm in patients 1, 3, and 4, and during dual chamber atrioventricular (AV) sequential pacing in patient 2. The white asterisk on the map of patient 2 denotes the pacing lead site as derived from CT. For each patient, the QRS duration (QRSd) is listed, followed by the calculated electrical dyssynchrony (ED) index. LA, left atrium; LV, left ventricle; RA, right atrium; RV, right ventricle. (*From* Silva JN, Ghosh S, Bowman TM, et al. Cardiac resynchronization therapy in pediatric congenital heart disease: insights from noninvasive electrocardiographic imaging. Heart Rhythm 2009;6(8):1181; with permission.)

therapy and had a brief period of improvement followed by quick decompensation. The patient went on to be listed as a status 1A for heart transplant (the highest status), but unfortunately died while awaiting transplant.

Pre-cardiac resynchronization therapy and post-cardiac resynchronization therapy electrocardiographic imaging patients

Patients 5 and 6 underwent ECGI activation isochronal mapping both before and after CRT.

The pre-CRT images were obtained to determine patient candidacy for CRT and potentially for targeted lead placement. The post-CRT images were obtained to determine response to CRT.

Patient 5 is a 6-year-old boy with congenitally corrected transposition of the great arteries. Past surgical intervention included the placement of a 16-mm homograft from the left ventricle to the pulmonary artery, which resulted in high-grade AV block, requiring the implantation of a dual chamber pacemaker by age 15 months. Pre-CRT ECGI was obtained (**Fig. 12**, top panel) and demonstrated that the patient had an ED of 36.4, indicative of severe dyssynchrony. Activation isochrones delineated an area of late activation in the posterolateral basilar region of the systemic right ventricle as a potential target for resynchronization lead. Postoperative CRT ECGI images were subsequently obtained under 5 conditions with the following ED indices: (1) CRT-OPT, ED of 21 ms, (2) CRT-NOM, ED of 29.3 ms, (3) PV-P (subpulmonary ventricular pacing only), ED of 36.4 ms, (4) SV-P (systemic ventricular pacing only), ED of 32.3 ms, and (5) SR (at this visit, the patient had intact conduction), ED of 23.4 ms. Interestingly, when the patient presented he had intact AV conduction that was able to be imaged by ECGI. This condition showed a normal ED index with a normal activation pattern. Given the intermittent nature of his AV conduction, he was mostly in a paced

Pre- and Post-CRT ECGI Activation-Isochrones in Patient #5

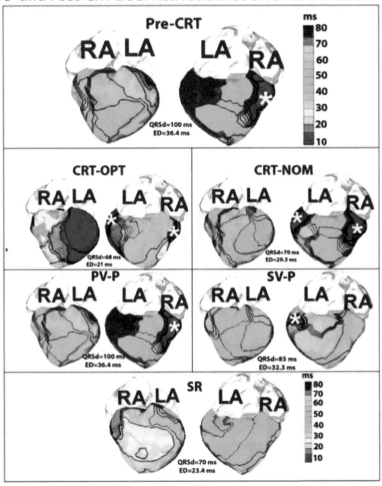

Fig. 12. The pre- and post-cardiac resynchronization therapy (CRT) activation electrocardiographic imaging (ECGI) maps from patient 5, shown in anterior and inferior projections. For each condition, the QRS duration (QRSd) is listed, followed by the calculated electrical dyssynchrony (ED) index. The epicardial pacing sites are marked by white asterisks. CRT-NOM, nominal CRT; CRT-OPT, optimal CRT; LA, left atrium; LV, left ventricle; PV-P, subpulmonary ventricular pacing only; RA, right atrium; RV, right ventricle; SV-P, systemic ventricular pacing only. (*From* Silva JN, Ghosh S, Bowman TM, et al. Cardiac resynchronization therapy in pediatric congenital heart disease: insights from noninvasive electrocardiographic imaging. Heart Rhythm 2009;6(8):1182; with permission.)

rhythm, and the condition CRT-OPT had a normal ED index as well, a significant improvement over single site ventricular pacing. Clinically, the patient had symptomatic improvement and was able to return to activities.

Patient 6 is an 8-year-old boy with hypoplastic left heart syndrome, mitral atresia, and double outlet right ventricle who had a dual chamber pacemaker implanted at 3 months of age for postoperative heart block (original ventricular pacing lead placed at the site of the white asterisk, **Fig. 13**). By age 8, the patient had developed symptoms of heart failure and was maximized on medical therapy. **Fig. 13** shows his ventricular activation maps imaged by ECGI. His pre-CRT maps show an ED index of 50 ms, which is severely abnormal. Additionally, the latest site of electrical

activation was identified (left anterior and inferior basal aspects of the single ventricle), and was the target site for epicardial lead implantation. Three months postoperatively, the patient underwent repeat ECGI studies under the following 4 conditions with the following ED indices: (1) CRT-OPT, ED of 27 ms, (2) CRT-NOM, ED of 29 ms, (3) ANT-P (anterior aspect of single ventricle), ED of 31 ms, and (4) POST-P (posterior aspect of the single ventricle), ED of 50 ms. CRT-OPT conditions yielded the most improved ED index, although it remained slightly abnormally prolonged. Single site ventricular pacing, from either the anterior or posterior aspects of the univentricle, yielded moderate to severely abnormal ED indices, respectively. Clinically, the patient was a CRT responder and improved with medical and

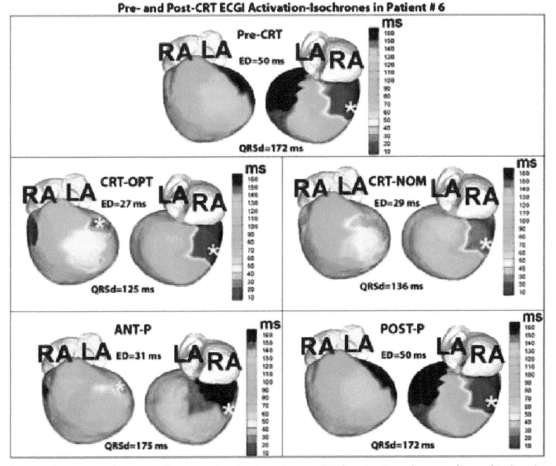

Fig. 13. The pre- and post-cardiac resynchronization therapy (CRT) activation electrocardiographic imaging (ECGI) maps from patient 6, shown in anterior and inferior projections. For each condition, the QRS duration (QRSd) is listed, followed by the calculated electrical dyssynchrony (ED) index. White asterisks denote sites of pacing leads. CRT-NOM, nominal CRT; CRT-OPT, optimal CRT; LA, left atrium; LV, left ventricle; PV-P, subpulmonary ventricular pacing only; RA, right atrium; RV, right ventricle; SV-P, systemic ventricular pacing only. (*From* Silva JN, Ghosh S, Bowman TM, et al. Cardiac resynchronization therapy in pediatric congenital heart disease: insights from noninvasive electrocardiographic imaging. Heart Rhythm 2009;6(8):1183; with permission.)

device therapy. This patient's poor clinical status before CRT may be partially explained by the severe dyssynchrony seen in his baseline paced rhythm.

Post-cardiac resynchronization therapy electrocardiographic imaging patients

Patients 7 and 8 underwent ECGI activation mapping after CRT only. Interestingly, these patients had similar underlying intracardiac anatomy.

Patient 7 is a 17-year-old girl with double inlet left ventricle, L-transposition of the great arteries, s/p fenestrated Fontan, and a dual chamber epicardial pacemaker for sinoatrial nodal dysfunction and second degree atrioventricular block. She underwent maximization of medical therapy as well as an upgrade from dual chamber to CRT pacing in 2006 for progressive heart failure symptoms. The second ventricular lead was empirically placed approximately 180° apart from the original ventricular pacing lead. Clinically, she had an improvement in her heart failure symptoms with medical and device therapy. ECGI ventricular activation isochronal maps were performed (**Fig. 14**) under 4 conditions with the following ED indices: (1) CRT-OPT, ED of 18.4 ms, (2) CRT-NOM, ED

of 21.2 ms, (3) ANT-P, ED of 32.8 ms, and (4) POST-P, ED of 34.7 ms. Single site ventricular pacing from either the anterior or posterior lead yielded abnormal ED indices as compared with CRT pacing, which nearly normalized the ED index.

Patient 8 is a 21-year-old woman with double inlet left ventricle and L-transposition of the great arteries, s/p fenestrated Fontan procedure, and a dual chamber epicardial pacemaker for postoperative heart block. She underwent upgrade from a dual chamber pacemaker to a CRT pacemaker with the second lead empirically implanted approximately 180° from the original lead. ECGI ventricular activation maps were constructed (**Fig. 15**) under 3 conditions with the following ED indices: (1) CRT-OPT, ED of 37.3 ms, (2) ANT-P, ED of 36.5 ms, and (3) POST-P, ED of 38.8 ms. Interestingly, these maps clearly show regions of slow conduction (crowded isochrones) and lines of conduction block (thick black lines) located on the anterior and posterior surfaces of the heart encompassing the ventricular pacing leads. This configuration left large swaths of the ventricular myocardium unpaced and therefore not resynchronized, which resulted

Post-CRT ECGI Activation-Isochrones in Patient # 7

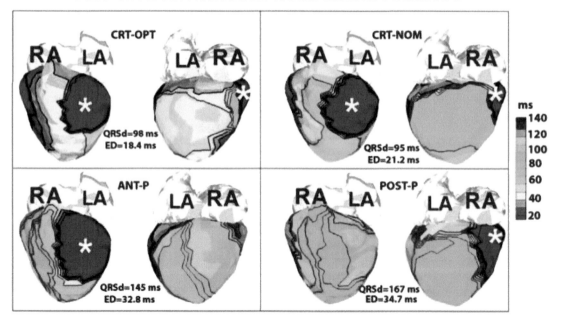

Fig. 14. The post-cardiac resynchronization therapy (CRT) activation electrocardiographic imaging (ECGI) maps from patient 7 are shown in anterior and inferior projections. For each condition, the QRS duration (QRSd) is listed, followed by the calculated electrical dyssynchrony (ED) index. White asterisks denote epicardial leads. CRT-NOM, nominal CRT; CRT-OPT, optimal CRT; LA, left atrium; LV, left ventricle; PV-P, subpulmonary ventricular pacing only; RA, right atrium; RV, right ventricle; SV-P, systemic ventricular pacing only. (*From* Silva JN, Ghosh S, Bowman TM, et al. Cardiac resynchronization therapy in pediatric congenital heart disease: insights from noninvasive electrocardiographic imaging. Heart Rhythm 2009;6(8):1184; with permission.)

Post-CRT ECGI Activation-Isochrones in Patient #8

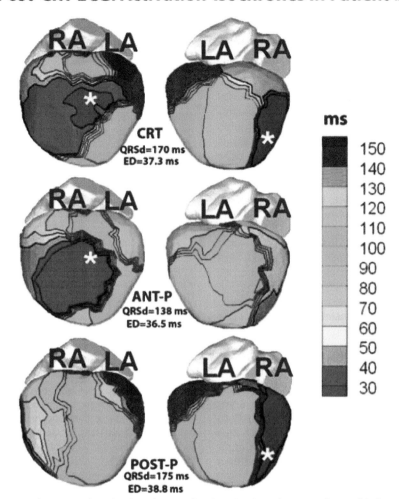

Fig. 15. The post-cardiac resynchronization therapy (CRT) activation electrocardiographic imaging (ECGI) maps from patient 8 are shown in anterior and inferior projections. For each condition, the QRS duration (QRSd) is listed, followed by the calculated electrical dyssynchrony (ED) index. White asterisks mark the location of epicardial pacing leads. ANT-P, anterior aspect of single ventricle; LA, left atrium; POST-P, posterior aspect of the single ventricle; RA, right atrium. (*From* Silva JN, Ghosh S, Bowman TM, et al. Cardiac resynchronization therapy in pediatric congenital heart disease: insights from noninvasive electrocardiographic imaging. Heart Rhythm 2009;6(8):1185; with permission.)

in persistent ED that did not improve with CRT-OPT pacing. Clinically, this patient was not a CRT responder and continued to have worsening heart failure symptoms. She eventually was listed for a cardiac transplant and was successfully transplanted.

Summary

ECGI provides an objective measure of dyssynchrony. If we were to make the assumption that electrical dyssynchrony precedes mechanical dyssynchrony, then identification of patients before CRT who have electrical dyssynchrony may help to reduce the number of CRT nonresponders by identifying those patients with normal ED.

The ED index is expected to be higher for those patients with regions of late ventricular activation, rather than those patients with generalized slow conduction. For example, patient 2 had a prolonged QRS duration of 125 ms, reflecting generalized slow conduction through the ventricular myocardium. However, ECGI demonstrated that the slow conduction was generalized throughout the myocardial mass, yielding a rather normal ED index of 20.5 ms. In contrast, patient 4 had a

QRS duration of 100 ms though ECGI activation maps demonstrated large areas of very late activation (dark blue) and a resultant abnormal ED index of 37 ms.

Site Selection for the Resynchronization Lead

Currently, there are no objective criteria for resynchronization lead placement. Often, epicardial resynchronization leads are placed approximately 180° apart on the epicardium. However, targeted site selection for the resynchonization lead is more likely to achieve resynchronization, as seen in patients 5 and 6. In these patients, the maps were shown to the operating surgeons to identify the general anatomic area for lead placement. ECGI provides an objective basis for the site selection.

ECGI helps to define the electrophysiologic substrate before implantation of the CRT. For example, patient 8 had a significantly abnormal electrophysiologic substrate with regions on slow conduction and lines of conduction block. CRT did not yield the desired clinical response in this patient. In this patient, one of the ventricular leads was placed adjacent to an area of slow conduction, leaving one half of the ventricular mass devoid of resynchonization pacing. Optimally, the CRT leads should be paced in areas to resynchronize large portions of the myocardium. Performing ECGI before CRT may help to better understand each patient's unique electrophysiologic substrate (regions of slow conduction, lines of block) before resynchronization lead placement.

Improvement in clinical response may be accompanied by more synchronized ventricular contraction and a lower ED index, as demonstrated by patients 5, 6, and 7.

SUMMARY

ECGI can be performed safely and effectively in the pediatric population. There is much to be learned mechanistically given the heterogeneity of pediatric substrates, including congenital heart disease patients. In addition, there may be clinically relevant data that may alter the way we take care of these young, ill patients. Future pediatric studies are needed to further our knowledge of these patient substrates.

REFERENCES

1. Ghosh S, Avari JN, Rhee RK, et al. Noninvasive electrocardiographic imaging (ECGI) of epicardial activation before and after catheter ablation of the accessory pathway in a patient with Ebstein anomaly. Heart Rhythm 2008;5(6):857–60.
2. Arruda MS, McClelland JH, Wang X, et al. Development and validation of an ECG algorithm for identifying accessory pathway ablation site in Wolff-Parkinson-White syndrome. J Cardiovasc Electrophysiol 1998; 9(1):2–12.
3. Ghosh S, Avari JN, Rhee EK, et al. Hypertrophic cardiomyopathy with preexcitation: insights from noninvasive electrocardiographic imaging (ECGI) and catheter mapping. J Cardiovasc Electrophysiol 2008; 19(11):1215–7.
4. Lipshultz SE, Sleeper LA, Towbin JA, et al. The incidence of pediatric cardiomyopathy in two regions of the United States. N Engl J Med 2003;348(17):1647–55.
5. Ghosh S, Rhee EK, Avari JN, et al. Cardiac memory in patients with Wolff-Parkinson-White syndrome: noninvasive imaging of activation and repolarization before and after catheter ablation. Circulation 2008;118(9):907–15.
6. Avari JN, Rhee EK. Cardiac resynchronization therapy for pediatric heart failure. Heart Rhythm 2008; 5(10):1476–8.

Distinct Localized Reentrant Drivers in Persistent Atrial Fibrillation Identified by Noninvasive Mapping
Relation to f-wave Morphology

Han S. Lim, MBBS, PhD, Nicolas Derval, MD,
Arnaud Denis, MD, Stephan Zellerhoff, MD,
Michel Haissaguerre, MD*

KEYWORDS

- Noninvasive mapping • Localized drivers • Persistent atrial fibrillation • Catheter ablation
- f-wave morphology

KEY POINTS

- Noninvasive mapping enables panoramic beat-to-beat mapping during atrial fibrillation (AF).
- Localized driving sources during persistent AF identified by noninvasive mapping correlate with distinct f-wave morphologies.
- Ablation of these driver regions results in prolongation of the AF cycle length and eventual termination of the arrhythmia.

CLINICAL HISTORY

The following case describes a 67-year-old man with persistent atrial fibrillation (AF) of 5 months' duration. The patient was referred for catheter ablation of persistent AF. The left atrium (LA) was dilated at 27 cm². Twelve-lead electrocardiogram (ECG) of the patient (**Fig. 1**A) showed dynamically changing f-wave patterns. There were 2 predominant f-wave patterns: the first was negative in the inferior leads, and the second was positive in the inferior leads.

NONINVASIVE MAPPING

A body vest comprising 252 electrodes was applied to the patient's torso to record surface potentials. The methodology is previously described in detail.[1] The patient underwent noncontrast computed tomography scan to obtain a 3-dimensional individualized geometry of the patient's left (LA) and right atria (RA). The exact locations of the body surface electrodes on the patient's torso in relation to the cardiac geometry were also acquired during this time. For patients who present in AF, noninvasive mapping may be performed at the bedside or in the electrophysiology laboratory.

Consecutive R-R pauses of greater than 1 second were recorded for analysis. The T-Q segments were selected to avoid QRST interference. Phase mapping algorithms were applied to identify reentrant

Disclosure: This work was supported through the Investment of the Future grant, ANR-10-IAHU-04, from the government of France through the Agence National de la Recherche. Dr. Haissaguerre is a stockowner in CardioInsight Inc., Cleveland, OH, USA.
IHU LIRYC, Electrophysiology and Heart Modeling Institute, Fondation Bordeaux Université, Bordeaux, France
* Corresponding author.
E-mail address: michel.haissaguerre@chu-bordeaux.fr

cardiacEP.theclinics.com

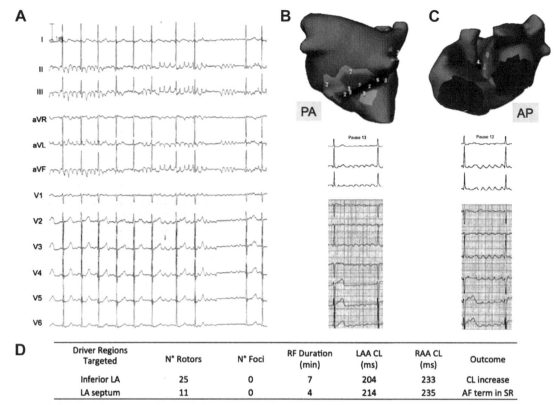

Driver Regions Targeted	N° Rotors	N° Foci	RF Duration (min)	LAA CL (ms)	RAA CL (ms)	Outcome
Inferior LA	25	0	7	204	233	CL increase
LA septum	11	0	4	214	235	AF term in SR

Fig. 1. (*A*) Twelve-lead ECG of the patient showed dynamically changing f-wave patterns. (*B, C*) Aggregated driver density maps of the left and right atria, with the posteroanterior (PA) view shown in panel B and antero-posterior (AP) view shown in panel C. Reentrant activity was observed in the inferior LA and the LA septum. Localized driver activity was observed to correlate with f-wave morphology. (*D*) Parameters of targeted driver regions.

activity. Reentrant activity was defined as a wave that is observed to fully rotate around a functional core on wave progression and was verified by sequential activation of local unipolar electrograms covering the local cycle length (CL) around the pivot point. An aggregated map summating all recorded reentrant driver activity is displayed in the top region of panels B (posteroanterior view of the LA and RA) and C (anteroposterior view of the LA and RA). To minimize false positives, reentrant driver activity was defined only when 2 or more fully rotated events were recorded.

The aggregated driver density map revealed 2 areas of concentrated reentrant driver activity, which are highlighted in orange in **Fig. 1**: (1) the inferior LA (panel B), and (2) the LA septum (panel C). There were no focal drivers observed. Interestingly, during recording windows wherein the corresponding f-wave was negative in the inferior leads on 12-lead ECG, reentrant driver activity was noted to arise from the inferior LA (recording pause 13, panel B). In contrast, when driver activity was noted to arise from the LA septum, the corresponding f-waves were positive in the inferior leads on surface ECG (recording pause 12, panel C).

PROCEDURAL DETAILS

The following catheters were used during the electrophysiological study for mapping and ablation: (1) a steerable decapolar catheter (5-mm interelectrode spacing; Xtrem, Sorin Medical, Montrouge, France) positioned in the coronary sinus; (2) an irrigated 3.5-mm tip quadripolar catheter (Thermocool; Biosense-Webster, Diamond Bar, CA, USA) for ablation; and (3) a 20-pole multispline mapping catheter (PentaRay; Biosense-Webster) in the LA or RA. Transseptal puncture was performed to gain access into the LA. Heparin was administered with a target activated clotting time of 250 to 300 seconds.

The mean AF CL was calculated by averaging greater than 30 consecutive beats using automated software (BARD Electrophysiology, Lowell, MA, USA) and was manually verified. The average LA appendage CL was 172 ms at baseline.

Based on the aggregated driver density map, the first driver region that was most prevalent was the inferior LA (total number of rotor rotations recorded during the recording period was 25). Point by point radiofrequency (RF) ablation was applied in this region, specifically at the sites where reentrant activity was identified.[2] Following 7 minutes of RF ablation at this first driver region, average AF CL increased from 172 ms to 204 ms in the LA and 233 ms in the RA (see **Fig. 1**D). The second driver region was the LA septum (total number of rotor rotations recorded = 11). Ablation was performed at this site, which resulted in progressive AF CL slowing to 214 ms in the LA, and 235 ms in the RA. Four minutes into ablation at this second driver region, AF terminated into sinus rhythm.

DISCUSSION

This case demonstrates the feasibility of noninvasive mapping to identify localized driving sources in persistent AF. In this particular case, persistent AF was driven by reentrant activity originating from 2 predominant sources: the inferior LA and the LA septum.

Noninvasive mapping was able to identify these 2 localized sources, which were spatially distinct. Single or multiple discrete sources during AF have been described in previous animal studies.[3,4] Temporally, reentrant activity was usually nonsustained, with most reentrant activity lasting 2 to 3 rotations.[2] However, with cumulative recording windows, reentrant activity was observed to recur at the same sites (panels B and C). Reentrant activity may be intermittent or coexist at different locations.[3] However, in this case, when the surface ECG demonstrated distinctly negative f-waves in the inferior leads, reentrant driver activity was observed to arise from the inferior LA (panel B). Conversely, during reentrant driver activity arising from the LA septum, surface f-waves were noted to be positive in the inferior leads. This case illustrates that different localized driver sources may be active at different times, and their activity may be detected by noninvasive mapping and correlated with surface f-wave morphology.

The extent of reentrant activity recorded at each driver site provided information on which site was more active. Ablation starting at the inferior LA (which recorded 25 reentrant rotations) significantly prolonged the AF CL. As previously demonstrated in computer models, AF CL progressively prolongs when there are less and less participating drivers.[5] Furthermore, a critical number of participating drivers need to be eliminated before the arrhythmia is no longer sustained.[5] In this case, with the elimination of the second driver, AF was terminated. The fact that AF CL significantly prolonged and AF terminated following ablation of these localized drivers suggested that they were active participants of the AF process. Total RF ablation time for this case was 11 minutes. In a recent study, catheter ablation of driver domains in persistent AF guided by noninvasive mapping significantly reduced the extent of ablation, while maintaining long-term outcomes compared with a conventional stepwise ablation cohort.[2]

SUMMARY

This case demonstrates the utility of noninvasive mapping in identifying localized driving sources in persistent AF. These localized sources are often multiple and are periodically active. Reentrant driver activity detected by noninvasive mapping from specific regions correlated with distinct f-wave morphologies. Elimination of these drivers by ablation resulted in progressive AF CL prolongation and termination of AF.

REFERENCES

1. Haissaguerre M, Hocini M, Shah AJ, et al. Noninvasive panoramic mapping of human atrial fibrillation mechanisms: a feasibility report. J Cardiovasc Electrophysiol 2013;24:711–7.
2. Haissaguerre M, Hocini M, Denis A, et al. Driver domains in persistent atrial fibrillation. Circulation 2014;130:530–8.
3. Skanes AC, Mandapati R, Berenfeld O, et al. Spatiotemporal periodicity during atrial fibrillation in the isolated sheep heart. Circulation 1998;98:1236–48.
4. Mandapati R, Skanes A, Chen J, et al. Stable microreentrant sources as a mechanism of atrial fibrillation in the isolated sheep heart. Circulation 2000;101:194–9.
5. Haissaguerre M, Lim KT, Jacquemet V, et al. Atrial fibrillatory cycle length: computer simulation and potential clinical importance. Europace 2007;9(Suppl 6):vi64–70.

Rotors in Patients with Persistent Atrial Fibrillation

Case Report of a Left Atrial Appendage Rotor Identified by a Novel Computational Mapping Algorithm Integrated into 3-Dimensional Mapping and Termination of Atrial Fibrillation with Ablation

Thomas Kurian, MD[a],*, Amit Doshi, MD[a], Paul Kessman, BS[b],
Bao Nguyen, BS[b], Jerome Edwards, BS, MBA[b],
Stephen Pieper, MD[a], Igor Efimov, PhD[c],
Ajit H. Janardhan, MD, PhD[b], Mauricio Sanchez, MD[a]

KEYWORDS

- Persistent atrial fibrillation • Panoramic AF mapping • Left atrial appendage • Ablation

KEY POINTS

- The cornerstone for catheter-based approaches to treat symptomatic paroxysmal atrial fibrillation (PAF) has historically been based on circumferential pulmonary vein isolation (PVI).
- The role of PVI in patients with persistent AF (PsAF) and long-standing PsAF (LsPAF) typically requires extensive ablation with a variety of approaches and techniques.
- Recent imaging modalities have been developed with the use of intracardiac baskets and high-density body surface electrodes allowing AF to be imaged in a panoramic field of view. These tools have provided insight into the mechanisms that maintain AF in patients with PsAF and LsPAF and identified AF drivers in the form of rotors and focal impulses.
- Targeting AF drivers using these technologies has recently been shown to reduce procedure times and improve outcomes in patients with PsAF and LsPAF.
- The left atrial appendage (LAA) has been shown to be an extrapulmonary source of AF; targeting sources within/around the LAA has resulted in termination of AF and improved AF outcomes.

Disclosures: T. Kurian, M. Sanchez, A. Doshi, B. Nguyen, P. Kessman, J. Edwards, and A.H. Janardhan have equity options/consulting agreements with CardioNXT, Inc. T. Kurian and J. Edwards are cofounders of CardioNXT and also hold positions on the company's board of directors.
[a] Division of Cardiac Electrophysiology, Mercy Heart & Vascular Center, St Louis, 625 South New Ballas Road, Suite 2030, St Louis, MO 63141, USA; [b] CardioNXT, Inc, 10955 Westmoor Drive, Westminster, CO 80021, USA; [c] Department of Biomedical Engineering, Washington University in St Louis, 360 Whitaker Hall, 1 Brookings Drive, St Louis, MO 63130, USA
* Corresponding author.
E-mail address: tkurian76@gmail.com

INTRODUCTION

Atrial fibrillation (AF) is the most common cardiac arrhythmia worldwide and is associated with increased risks of stroke, heart failure, hospitalizations, and mortality.[1,2] Catheter-based treatment has been historically based on targeting the triggers of AF, which are thought to be mainly located within the pulmonary veins (PVs).[3] This approach has had success in the treatment of paroxysmal AF (PAF); however, its role in persistent AF (PsAF) and long-standing PsAF (LsPAF) has been limited, largely because of poorly understood mechanisms of the driving influences that maintain AF.[4]

Recent technological advancements have provided further insight into mechanisms driving PsAF and LsPAF with the use of intracardiac baskets and high-density body-surface electrodes, creating an opportunity for panoramic imaging to elucidate the mechanism that maintain AF in patients.[5,6] Using these novel technologies, AF drivers have been identified and described as rotors and focal Impulses. With a panoramic field of view of human AF, drivers of AF can be targeted with catheter ablation. Using these technologies, an AF driver-directed approach guiding ablation in PsAF and LsPAF has produced promising initial results potentially reducing procedure times and improving outcomes in this difficult-to-treat patient population.[7,8]

The left atrial appendage (LAA) is traditionally thought of as the major source of thromboembolism in patients with AF, which can result in disabling strokes.[9] In addition, recent studies have revealed the LAA to be a source contributing to the initiation and possible maintenance of AF.[10]

CASE REPORT
Clinical History

Here we describe a 66-year-old white man with a history of hypertension, diabetes mellitus, and obstructive sleep with PsAF who underwent ablation with pulmonary vein isolation (PVI) and Linear Ablation. He was noted to have depressed left ventricular function by transthoracic echocardiography revealing an ejection fraction of 45%. Despite adequate rate control, he continued to report symptoms of fatigue and dyspnea on exertion, which he correlated with the onset of his AF. He initially underwent antiarrhythmic drug load with dofetilide and cardioversion but was noted to have early recurrence of AF (ERAF). Given his symptoms, he was offered a catheter-based ablation approach with PVI and linear ablation using radiofrequency ablation. Transesophageal echocardiography before the procedure

was noted for a mildly dilated left atrium (LA) with a septal to lateral wall dimension of 4.9 cm.

Research Protocol

This patient was a participant in an Institutional Review Board–approved study at Mercy Heart and Vascular Hospital (St Louis, MO) evaluating a novel computational mapping algorithm (CMA; CardioNXT, Westminster, CO) that recreates 3-dimenional (3D) panoramic unipolar maps with the collection of local near-field electrograms with circular mapping catheters (LASSO, Biosense Webster, Diamond Bar, CA) in a sequential fashion during LA geometry creation while the patient is in AF. A novel pattern-recognition algorithm derived from the CMA analyzed local near-field and far-field signals and detected correlations in AF allowing for the recreation of 3D panoramic unipolar AF maps.

Local unipolar signals were then evaluated in the context of their identified and reassigned locations within the 3D LA geometry created during the procedure and analyzed with conduction vector analyses. Conduction vectors in AF were created based on the relationship between identified unipolar signals obtained with the circular duodecapolar catheters and integrated within the 3D LA map. Local unipolar signals were then filtered and processed with CMA to identify the drivers of AF in the form of rotors and focal impulses.

In addition, further evaluation of local electrograms was performed, including continuous fractionated atrial electrogram (CFAE) analysis and mean voltage in AF. CFAE and mean voltage in AF were subsequently correlated in the context of identified AF drivers. Analysis was performed off-line after the procedure, with rhythm changes that were noted during the case evaluated in relation to the (1) CMA-identified drivers and (2) incidental ablation during the procedure with standard PVI and linear ablation.

Procedural Details

The patient was brought to the electrophysiology laboratory in a fasting state, intubated, and sedated under general anesthesia. Catheters were introduced via the femoral veins. Double transseptal access was guided by intracardiac ultrasound and fluoroscopy. Heparin was administered to maintain an ACT greater than 350 throughout the case once transseptal access was obtained. Standard catheters were placed, including a linear decapolar catheter in the coronary sinus (Inquiry, St Jude Medical, St Paul, Minnesota) and a circular duodecapolar catheter (LASSO) in the LA. Detailed 3D electroanatomic

LA maps were created with a 3D mapping system (Ensite Velocity, St Jude Medical, St Paul, Minnesota) using circular duodecapolar catheters in patients while in AF. Local electrograms were recorded for 30-second intervals throughout the LA to ensure adequate data collection for off-line analysis with CMA.

Ablation was performed in a temperature control mode at 20 to 40 W with a 3.5-mm tip irrigated catheter (Thermocool, Biosense Webster) with lower power used on the posterior wall/LAA. This patient presented in AF, and the aforementioned AF mapping protocol was pursued with subsequent standard-of-care PVI and linear ablation. PVI was pursued with wide area circumferential ablation performed initially. However, given the perpetuation of AF despite confirmation of PV

isolation, linear ablation was performed with a roofline connecting the right superior PV (RSPV) to the left superior PV (LSPV) and a mitral isthmus line connecting the left inferior PV (LIPV) to the mitral annulus. Despite these efforts, no evidence of organization of AF was observed; further unsuccessful ablation was pursued with linear ablation connecting the right inferior PV to the mitral annulus. Ablation was then pursued in the right atrium (RA) without obvious organization of AF. Finally, the LAA was interrogated and noted to have continuous electrical activation with notable fractionation (**Fig. 1**). Given that the (1) local signals were noted to be of high frequency with continuous activation and (2) the inability to terminate AF despite extensive ablation, radiofrequency ablation (RFA) was performed in the LAA

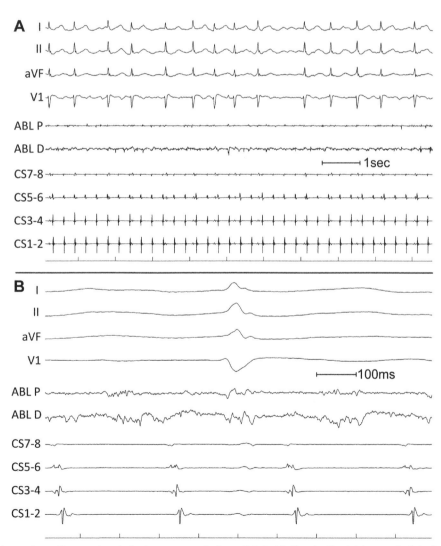

Fig. 1. Prolonged, continuous local electrograms noted on distal ablation in the LAA as noted during mapping while in AF noted at low (*A*) and high (*B*) sweep speeds in AF.

at 20 W/40° targeting local potentials. This procedure ultimately terminated AF into normal sinus rhythm (NSR).

COMPUTATIONAL MAPPING ALGORITHM ANALYSIS

Postprocedure analysis with CMA of local unipolar raw data integrated into a 3D panoramic AF map was performed before ablation. CMA identified 4 drivers of AF. There were 4 rotors; no focal impulses were identified in this case. Of the 4 rotors identified, 2 rotors were noted to be stable but migratory in space within the regions identified via CMA (**Fig. 2**; note LAA and LSPV, highlighted yellow) and noted to recur in multiple reconstructed AF maps with respect to time. The 2 remaining rotors were noted to be unstable in nature (**Fig. 3**; LAA and the anterior aspect of left-sided PVs, highlighted black).

Fast Fourier transform (FFT) of coronary sinus (CS) electrograms was analyzed and noted for change from 5.8 Hz to 5.5 Hz with isolation of the left-side PVs; however, there was no organization of AF. There was no change in FFT noted with isolation of the right-sided PVs. Rotors that were noted to be stable in nature but migratory seemed to move along voltage transition zones when superimposed over a voltage map created in AF during LA geometry creation. Voltage transition zones were defined as a change in voltage of greater the 0.23 mV between 2 adjacent areas within the LA. Low voltage in AF was assigned to local unipolar intracardiac electrograms of 0.3 mV or less. The unstable rotors identified did not seem to be associated with *voltage transition* zones ($\Delta V <0.23$ mV) in AF but were noted to occur in *low voltage* zones (<0.3 mV). Ablation that was performed in the LAA during the case was noted to incidentally transect

the migratory stable rotor that was identified in the LAA, resulting in the organization of AF and ultimately termination into NSR (**Fig. 4**).

SUMMARY/DISCUSSION

Ablation within and/or isolation of the LAA has been previously described and pursued by certain groups as part of a catheter-based approach for the treatment of AF. Using a novel CMA, the authors describe a unique case in which extensive linear ablation was performed in the LA/RA without organization of AF. Ultimately, ablation guided by targeting local prolonged fractionated electrograms within the LAA terminated AF with conversion to NSR. CMA data collection and postprocessing analysis for this case was notable for having identified drivers of AF in the form of 4 rotors. Further classification and characterization revealed 2 stable rotors and 2 unstable rotors. The stable rotors were located within LAA and within the LSPV. The 2 unstable rotors identified were located within the LAA (posterior to the identified stable rotor in the LAA) and on the anterior aspect of the LSPV/LIPV.

Thus far, in the authors' series of patients, the LAA typically is noted to be a homogeneous high-voltage region as compared with the rest of the LA when in AF (**Fig. 5**A). Rotors and focal impulses from the authors' patient series thus far have also been noted to primarily exist along voltage transition zones (see **Fig. 5**B). In this case, however, the authors found notably lower voltages during AF identified in the LAA with (1) an identified rotor and (2) a voltage transition zone along which the rotor seemed to migrate. Incidental ablation in the region of the identified stable rotor identified by the CMA in the LAA was noted to terminate AF to NSR. Clinically, the patient has had a recurrence

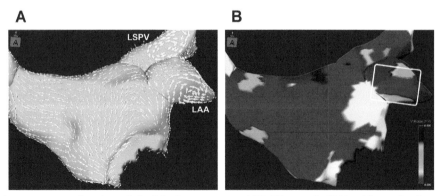

Fig. 2. (*A*) An anteroposterior view of the LA of reconstructed 3D AF map via CMA with conduction vector analysis map revealing 2 out of 4 identified (*yellow arrows*). (*B*) Voltage map in AF with patchy voltage transition zones in LAA as measured in AF (red <0.3 mV, magenta >1.0 mV.) The highlighted rotor within the LAA seems to migrate along the voltage transition zone noted within the LAA when viewed in multiple phases.

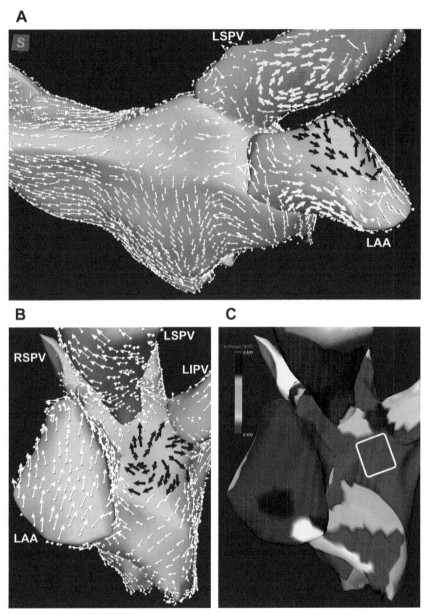

Fig. 3. (*A–C*) Four rotors were identified, with 2 stable rotors noted to repeat in multiple AF maps (*yellow arrows*) within the anterior aspect of LAA and the LSPV. Two unstable rotors (*black arrows*) were noted within the posterior part of the LAA and at the anterior aspect of the left-sided veins. These rotors were noted to occur infrequently in multiple AF maps evaluated and did not seem to occur near areas of voltage transition.

of atypical atrial flutter but has not had any evidence of recurrent AF.

This case is a unique example of a dramatic conversion of AF to NSR with ablation within the LAA guided by local electrograms and highlights the potential use of imaging modalities, such as CMA (CardioNXT), to identify drivers of AF in the context of 3D mapping systems. Previous studies have suggested that the LAA may contribute to the initiation and maintenance of AF, and targeting the LAA either focally or with LAA isolation was noted

to have improved outcomes with catheter ablation.[10] This case illustrates mechanistically, with identified drivers of AF located within the appendage, why this approach may be beneficial in certain cases.

Technological modalities that enable panoramic mapping of AF are providing clinicians with a new ability to evaluate AF and identify organized drivers in the form of rotors and focal impulses that perpetuate AF. Ultimately, this may provide clinicians with the ability to quickly identify regions

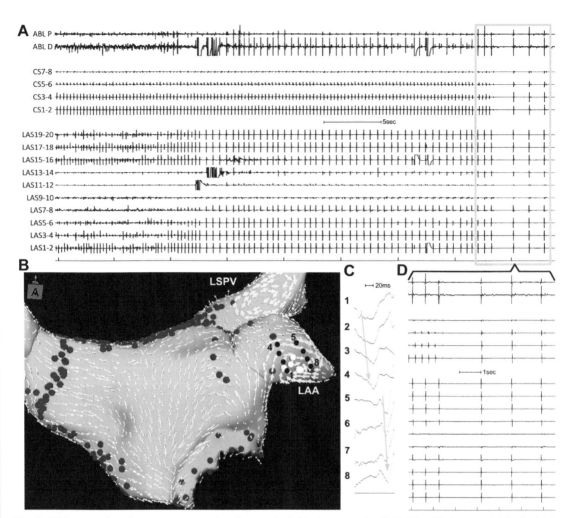

Fig. 4. (*A*) Intracardiac electrograms noted at the onset of ablation near the CMA-identified rotor within the LAA. Prolonged, continuous, and fractionated electrograms were noted on the distal ablation located within the LAA before RFA. (*B*) CMA identified a rotor noted to be within the LAA with ablation points noted to incidentally transect the rotor with AF termination corresponding to the highlighted ablation points (*white dots*). Red dots correspond with previous ablation points with PVI / Linear ablation. (*C*) Black dots in LAA represent points from integrated unipolar EGM in LAA derived from CMA highlighting local unipolar EGM around rotor core (*D*) AF is noted to organize and eventually terminate to NSR with RFA at this site.

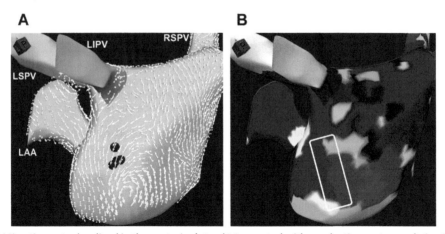

Fig. 5. (*A*) Migrating rotor localized in the posterior lateral LA as noted with conduction vector analysis with CMA integrated into 3D LA map. The rotor is noted to migrate along a voltage transition zone created from a voltage map in AF as denoted in (*B*) and classified as a migratory stable rotor as noted in multiple AF maps evaluated to migrate along the axis of the voltage transition zone. Rotor trajectory is noted with black dots as noted in multiple CMA-derived AF maps. Yellow arrows highlight identified rotor via conduction vector analysis with green dots representing rotor core.

within the atria driving AF, providing a platform to better understand the cause and mechanisms of AF maintenance and provide a more targeted catheter-based therapy for AF treatment.

REFERENCES

1. Wattigney WA, Mensah GA, Croft JB. Increasing trends in hospitalization for atrial fibrillation in the United States, 1985 through 1999: implications for primary prevention. Circulation 2003;108(6):711.
2. Stewart S, Hart CL, Hole DJ, et al. A population-based study of the long-term risks associated with atrial fibrillation: 20-year follow-up of the Renfrew/Paisley study. Am J Med 2002;113(5):359.
3. Haissaguerre M, Jais P, Shah DC, et al. Spontaneous initiation of atrial fibrillation by ectopic beats originating in the pulmonary veins. N Engl J Med 1998;339(10):659.
4. Wokhlu A, Hodge DO, Monahan KH, et al. Long-term outcome of atrial fibrillation ablation: impact and predictors of very late recurrence. J Cardiovasc Electrophysiol 2010;21(10):1071.
5. Narayan SM, Krummen DE, Rappel WJ. Clinical mapping approach to diagnose electrical rotors and focal impulse sources for human atrial fibrillation. J Cardiovasc Electrophysiol 2012;23(5):447.
6. Cuculich PS, Wang Y, Lindsay BD, et al. Noninvasive characterization of epicardial activation in humans with diverse atrial fibrillation patterns. Circulation 2010;122(14):1364.
7. Narayan SM, Krummen DE, Shivkumar K, et al. Treatment of atrial fibrillation by the ablation of localized sources: CONFIRM (Conventional Ablation for Atrial Fibrillation With or Without Focal Impulse and Rotor Modulation) trial. J Am Coll Cardiol 2012; 60(7):628.
8. Haassaguerre M, Hocini M, Denis A, et al. Driver domains in persistent atrial fibrillation. Circulation 2014; 130(7):530–8.
9. Reddy VY, Doshi SK, Sievert H, et al. Percutaneous left atrial appendage closure for stroke prophylaxis in patients with atrial fibrillation: 2.3-year follow-up of the PROTECT AF (Watchman Left Atrial Appendage System for Embolic Protection in Patients with Atrial Fibrillation) trial. Circulation 2013; 127(6):720.
10. Di Biase L, Burkhardt JD, Mohanty P, et al. Left atrial appendage: an underrecognized trigger site of atrial fibrillation. Circulation 2010;122(2):109.

Moving?

Make sure your subscription moves with you!

To notify us of your new address, find your **Clinics Account Number** (located on your mailing label above your name), and contact customer service at:

Email: journalscustomerservice-usa@elsevier.com

800-654-2452 (subscribers in the U.S. & Canada)
314-447-8871 (subscribers outside of the U.S. & Canada)

Fax number: 314-447-8029

Elsevier Health Sciences Division
Subscription Customer Service
3251 Riverport Lane
Maryland Heights, MO 63043

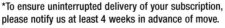

ELSEVIER

Printed and bound by CPI Group (UK) Ltd, Croydon, CR0 4YY

03/10/2024

01040382-0014